PRAISE FOR *Think Like a Pancreas*

"This book is an interesting read that utilizes humor and practical approaches to address the complex topic of managing diabetes with insulin. Touching on many of the everyday topics everyone taking insulin needs to master, it provides an organized and systematic approach to demystify the complexities of insulin and glucose regulation."

—*Diabetes Source*

"*Think Like a Pancreas* would make an idea gift for a loved one who is starting insulin therapy. Even those of us who have been taking insulin for years would do well to keep a copy on hand."

—*Diabetes Health*

"A thorough guide to the factors that go into optimal blood glucose control."

—*Diabetes Exercise and Sports Association* newsletter

"*In Think Like a Pancreas*, Gary Scheiner, a certified diabetes educator, walks the walk and talks the talk of mimicking the organ's finer functions…This is definitely a worthwhile read for patients and professionals who want enhanced knowledge, in order to truly 'think like a pancreas.'"

—*Voice of the Diabetic*

"Gary Scheiner knows as much about diabetes as most endocrinologists and he has translated his knowledge and experience into a well-written, easy-to-read treatise on diabetes. A must-read for anyone with an interest in diabetes—most importantly patients and their families."

—STEVEN B. NAGELBERG, MD, clinical endocrinologist

"*Think Like a Pancreas* is delightful, unique, comprehensive, and detail oriented. The writing style is easy to follow. It will enlighten and educate for sure. Great work, Gary."

—PAULA HARPER, founder and president of
the Diabetes Exercise and Sports Association

"Gary Scheiner offers the missing "manual" designed to benefit every patient with diabetes who wishes not only to optimize his/her self-care, but also to comprehend all the forces that work against easily achieving this lofty goal. He offers guidance, expertise, and a first-hand understanding of what it means to have to "think like a pancreas."

—RENEE BERNETT, mother of a child with type 1 diabetes
and member of the Juvenile Diabetes Research
Foundation's Lay Review Committee

"*Think Like a Pancreas* is the most helpful guide that I've encountered about the intricacies of using insulin. Gary Scheiner speaks as one of us—someone who's lived with diabetes for nearly twenty years—and is able to translate sophisticated scientific concepts into clear laymen's terms. His humor is motivational and his understanding of the frustrations that can come with using insulin is truly encouraging. Though I've taken insulin on a daily basis for over twenty-three years, *Think Like a Pancreas* has opened my eyes to many new nuances that will surely help me—and countless other people with diabetes—in my quest for tight blood sugar control."

—GABRIELLE KAPLAN-MAYER, author of
Insulin Pump Therapy Demystified,
www.insulinpumpbook.com

Think Like a Pancreas

A Practical Guide to Managing Diabetes with Insulin

GARY SCHEINER, MS, CDE

Foreword by Barry Goldstein, MD, PhD

Da Capo
LIFE
LONG

A Member of the Perseus Books Group

Set in 12 point Granjon by the Perseus Books Group

Cataloging-in-Publication data for this book
is available from the Library of Congress.

ISBN: 978-1-56924-436-4

Published by Da Capo Press
A Member of the Perseus Books Group
www.dacapopress.com

Da Capo Press books are available at special discounts for bulk
purchases in the U.S. by corporations, institutions, and other organizations.
For more information, please contact the Special Markets Department at the
Perseus Books Group, 2300 Chestnut Street, Suite 200, Philadelphia,
PA, 19103, or call (800) 810-4145, extension 5000, or e-mail
special.markets@perseusbooks.com.

15 14 13 12 11

To MJ, Bumble Bee, Naked Boy, and Butterbean

Contents

The information in this book is intended to help readers make informed decisions about their health and the health of their loved ones. It is not intended to be a substitute for treatment by or the advice and care of a professional health care provider. While the authors and publisher have endeavored to ensure that the information presented is accurate and up to date, they shall not be held responsible for loss or damage of any nature suffered as a result of reliance on any of this book's contents or any errors or omissions herein.

Foreword

By Dr. Barry Goldstein

DURING MY OWN TRAINING in clinical diabetes at the Joslin Diabetes Center in Boston, Elliott P. Joslin, an early pioneer of patient care and insulin therapy, was often quoted as describing how important it was for patients to learn about their diabetes not only from physicians but also from other patients and teachers. This has certainly been true to the present day. Watching the many positive interactions among people with diabetes and their nurses and educators has strongly influenced my own approach to the management of this disease. The role of the physician is to give therapeutic advice and general medical care and to screen for the many potential complications of diabetes and treat such complications if they arise. The practical issues that patients with diabetes confront on a daily basis, however, require a more grassroots approach.

In this comprehensive and very practical guide to the management of diabetes with insulin therapy, Gary Scheiner has offered the best of two worlds: not only is he a seasoned patient who takes meticulous care of his own diabetes, but he is also an accomplished and knowledgeable certified diabetes educator and exercise physiologist. The reader has a lot to gain by sharing Gary's own experiences and his wealth of practical management guidelines.

There is no question in my mind that a physician's best patient is one who is well-informed with up-to-date and practical information. Patients need to understand the physiology of diabetes and the influences of daily activities, diet, and exercise to fine-tune their insulin therapy. *Think Like a Pancreas* presents this information in a very readable manner and is a very useful and informative resource.

Health professionals and patients alike need to accept the fact that bringing glucose levels as close to normal as possible will help delay or altogether prevent the onset of most of the complications of diabetes. As we strive for this goal, we also wish that our patients can lead as normal and fulfilling lives as possible. Since this book will clearly help our friends, family members, and patients to achieve success in living with diabetes, I congratulate Gary on his achievement and hope that this book is widely used.

—Barry J. Goldstein, MD, PhD

Professor of Medicine and of Biochemistry
and Molecular Pharmacology

Director, Division of Endocrinology,
Diabetes and Metabolic Diseases

Jefferson Medical College of Thomas Jefferson University
Philadelphia

Preface

I BELIEVE THAT PEOPLE with diabetes are an intelligent and motivated bunch, capable of making sound decisions when given appropriate guidance and training. After all, to *Think Like a Pancreas*, people with diabetes have to be the ones doing the thinking!

The discovery of insulin gave us the ability to live with diabetes. But today, we want to do more than just *survive*. We want to *thrive*. And we have that opportunity if we *Think Like a Pancreas*. That means:

- utilizing the latest diabetes technologies and resources;

- setting up an insulin program conducive to your lifestyle, with a basal and bolus component;

- fine-tuning the basal insulin levels so that blood sugars are fairly stable between meals and during sleep;

- matching bolus insulin to the carbohydrate content of meals;

- adjusting boluses based on blood sugar levels and physical activity;

- analyzing records to find the causes of high and low readings, and making appropriate adjustments;

- taking reasonable steps to avoid extreme high and low blood sugars; and

- maintaining a positive, aggressive attitude toward blood sugar control.

I myself have been living with type 1 diabetes since 1986—I'll tell you more about my story in chapter 1—and I've been a certified diabetes educator since 1993. With *Think Like a Pancreas* I share with you everything I've learned professionally, as well as personally, about managing diabetes with insulin. Please note that the words and phrases which appear in **boldface** are defined in the glossary starting on page 211. I hope this book goes a long way to helping you manage your diabetes to the very best of your ability. And please don't hesitate to call on me personally for additional guidance.

—Gary Scheiner, MS, CDE
Integrated Diabetes Services
333 E. Lancaster Ave., Suite 204
Wynnewood, PA 19096
610-642-6055
fax: 610-642-8046
e-mail: garyscheiner@prodigy.net
www.integrateddiabetes.com

1 introduction

What's the Dang-Diddly Point?[1]

So, YOU HAVE DIABETES and take insulin. What could be simpler? How about predicting the stock market? The weather? The next five World Series winners?

By now you have discovered one common truism about managing diabetes with insulin: It ain't that simple. But . . . what's that? You already have a doctor who is taking care of your diabetes? That's just swell. In this age of assembly-line health care dictated by third-party managed care organizations, most physicians are limited in the amount of time they can spend with their patients. After taking vitals, reviewing histories and lab results, performing physical exams, ordering new lab work, and writing prescriptions, precious little time is available for your physician to sit down with you to teach you the finer points of living with diabetes and controlling your blood sugar levels. It's not from a lack of desire; most physicians I know are talented, motivated, caring people who wish they had the time and resources to do more for their patients.

Don't get me wrong. Your physician still plays a very important role in overseeing and directing your diabetes care. He or she

[1] with apologies to Ned Flanders of *The Simpsons*

should be viewed as an expert adviser who oversees your care rather than as the person who should micromanage every aspect of your disease. And it is *your* disease.

Diabetes forces us, as patients, to make countless important decisions every day. The time is now to learn how to do a better job of self-managing your diabetes, with your physician's guidance and input. With new insulins, insulin delivery devices, dosing formulas, dietary plans and monitoring systems, just about anyone can—and *should*—learn how to manage blood sugar levels effectively.

Gone are the days when your doctor gives you a fixed insulin dose and asks you to adjust your life to match the insulin. You can manage your diabetes with insulin and live a perfectly normal, varied life, doing the things you like to do when you like to do them—*if* you know what you're doing. The purpose of this book is to do just that: to teach you how to match your insulin to your body's ever-changing needs. In other words, to Think like pancreas.

My personal story of life with diabetes provides a good example.

My Story

It was two o'clock in the afternoon on a typically hot, muggy summer day in Sugarland, Texas (No, I'm not making this up. The irony is just unbelievable.). After spending half the summer sucking down cold drinks and the other half peeing them out, I decided it was time to see the family doctor.

I hardly knew this doctor. My family had moved to Sugarland just a year prior (I grew up in central New Jersey), but I had had about all I could take. My energy was almost gone, and there was no way the Houston summer could have caused me to lose all that weight (I had gone from 155 pounds to 117). The last straw came when my belt would not tighten enough to keep my pants from falling down. Then I saw an episode of *M*A*S*H* in which a chopper pilot with diabetes had the same symptoms I had, so I figured I'd better get myself checked out.

It was only a 10-minute drive from our house to the doctor's office, so I was able to make it with just one pit stop to use a gas station restroom. That summer, I learned where all the best public restrooms were along the I-59 corridor in southwest Houston. When I got to the doctor's office, I put *on* my glasses (miraculously, I was able to see road signs *without* my glasses for the first time in 10 years), wiped off the steam created by the 10,000% humidity, and prepared myself for the worst.

After a quick physical exam, blood test, and urinalysis, the doctor came back in and said nonchalantly, "Gary, I've got good news and I've got bad news. The bad news is that you have diabetes, and you're going to have it the rest of your life."

I have no idea what the good news was, because I stopped listening at that point. The first syllable from "diabetes" stuck in my head like a knife. What the heck does diabetes *mean?* About all I knew was that it had something to do with blood, that it could make people really sick, and that it wasn't going to go away. Ever.

I remember him telling me that my blood sugar level was 613, and that that was 6 times the normal level. I also remember him saying that I would have to take shots and be very careful of what I ate. The thought of giving myself shots was one thing. But limit what I eat? Was he *crazy?* I was an active 18-year-old with the metabolism of a small country. The very thought of not being able to eat whatever I wanted whenever I wanted made me hungrier than ever.

So, off I went to an endocrinologist at a fancy high-rise in downtown Houston. Keep in mind that the year was 1985 and there were no HMOs yet, so getting in to see a specialist was relatively simple.

"You are lucky to be diagnosed now," explained the endocrinologist. "We have come a long way in the treatment of diabetes. I bet that in 5 or 10 years, your diabetes will be cured."

That was 18 years ago.

The endocrinologist had me meet with a nurse, who taught me the "basics" about diabetes. I discovered what insulin is and why it is important. I learned about the importance of controlling blood sugar levels, and why the high blood sugars I had been experiencing all summer had turned me into a human sieve. She taught me how food and exercise affect blood sugars.

Finally, I was instructed on how to inject insulin. Forget the oranges, pillows, and teddy bears. I gave myself my very first injection, right in the stomach. It hurt—probably because I had almost no fat left on my body, and the syringe needles were much thicker and longer than they are today. But mostly it hurt because I was tense and overwhelmed at the thought of sticking needles in myself for the rest of my life.

I was also given a bottle of test strips and taught about blood sugar testing. No meter. Just test strips. These strips had a big square box on them (about the size of a Chicklet) that had to be covered with blood, blotted, then timed before matching the color of the box to the color chart on the bottle. Pale blue meant you were 40–70 mg/dl. Light blue, 70–100. Ocean blue, 100–125. Aqua-blue, 125–150. Just plain aqua, 150–200. Aqua-green, 200–250. Sea green, 250–350. Green, 350–450. Brownish green, look out. In other words, determining your precise blood sugar level required an advanced degree in fine arts with a major in color differentiation.

The bottle of test strips came with a medieval torture device called an "Auto-Let." The Auto-Let had a small disposable platform with a hole, where you placed the victim . . . er . . . I mean, your finger. A disposable 25-gauge lancet was placed in the firing mechanism, which swung around at high speed like a pendulum to stab your finger and make it bleed. I called it "The Guillotine."

Then I met with a dietitian—a tiny middle-aged woman who taught me the fine art of the "exchange" diet.

"You really don't have to change what you eat that much," she told me. "You just have to be careful not to eat too many concentrated sweets, fats, or very large portions of anything." Not change what I eat? Apparently, she had no idea who she was talking to.

I can still remember the "generous" 2,500 calorie exchange diet—chock-full of fruits, vegetables, meats, and starches. Oh, how I hated that piece of paper. I was hungry constantly. The exchange system meant that everything I ate had to be placed in a category, and that I could only eat so many things from each category at each meal and snack. Talk about sapping the fun out of eating!

My first "exchange diet" meal looked so puny on the plate. And there were no seconds, thirds, fourths, etc. I was hungry all day long.

The first week or two were really rough. Even after starving myself and doing everything I was asked to do, the stupid test strips kept turning aqua-blue instead of sea green, or maybe it was the other way around. Who cares? I cried a lot those first couple of weeks. My mom told me that my dad, normally an unemotional guy, had cried, too, and that he wished that it was him, and not me, who got diabetes.

The insulin program I was placed on didn't make things any easier: NPH and Regular, at breakfast and dinner. The Regular would peak in about 2 hours and last about 6; the NPH would peak in 6 hours and last about 12. Everyone at the endocrinologist's office kept telling me the same thing: "You can live a normal life, as long as you do things according to your insulin." Basically, that meant that I would have to eat certain things at certain times of day; exercise (with caution) at certain times of day; sleep only at certain times because of the need to take shots at specific times; and test my blood sugar at certain times. What could be more normal than that?

Back in 1985, two shots a day was the norm. So was making your life conform to your insulin program. But things did improve over time. I was given a "sliding scale" for my insulin, which was a good thing, because I was rarely "ocean blue." I probably had as many lows as I had highs, so my **glycosylated hemoglobin** levels showed a decent average; usually in the 6–7% range. But the low blood sugars were becoming more frequent and more severe, especially during the night. My doctor at college suggested that I move my dinnertime NPH to bedtime. While that helped cut down on the nighttime lows, I started having more lows before lunch. Oy vey.

Soon after my diagnosis, I purchased my first blood glucose meter—a Glucometer, to be exact. It weighed about a pound and was the size of a sandwich (but without the onion smell). The testing procedure is still etched in my brain: Guillotine, then squeeze out a big "hanging" drop of blood, dab the big box on the strip, start the counter, wait 1 minute, blot the strip and insert it in the meter, press the button again, and wait 90 seconds for that 58 or 314mg/dl to appear. (Just once, wouldn't you like to see a meter advertisement where the reading on the screen wasn't so *perfect*?)

That meter lasted about a year. Then Lifescan came out with its One Touch meters, and I jumped to get one. Imagine—no blotting, a round test area, and only 45 seconds from stick to result! I was in hypoglycemic heaven. It didn't do much for my control, but I did have an extra five minutes a day to spend doing things other than waiting for my test results.

That meter got a lot of use through college (I went to Washington University in St. Louis). Before dinner, my roommates used to gather in the common room to wager on my blood sugar level. Everyone threw a dollar on the table; closest guess took the loot. Some of them became pretty adept at the whole diabetes thing: they would ask questions like "What did you eat for lunch?" and "Did you work out this afternoon?" Talk about "getting by with a little help from my friends." It was lighthearted stuff like that that kept me from getting down about my diabetes.

Despite the technological improvements, I was still plagued by frequent high and low readings. Anyone with diabetes knows how those blood sugar swings make you feel—chronically fatigued and frustrated. Exercise was one thing that helped me keep a positive attitude. I had always been into sports, but after being diagnosed with diabetes, my passion and commitment to fitness soared to a whole new level. Every day, I would be getting some form of exercise. If there wasn't anybody to play basketball or racquetball with, I would be at the gym working out, riding my bike around the park, or jumping rope in the lounge to the beat of Motown music. Exercising made me feel like I was still strong, fit, and in control of my own health, despite having diabetes.

Unfortunately, the emotional "high" I got from exercise was often followed by a serious low blood sugar. One month into my first job out of college, I showed up for work in a complete mental stupor. Some days, I couldn't even remember getting dressed or driving in to work. It's amazing that I never crashed into a tree buck-naked. To make matters worse, I was no longer getting symptoms that a low blood sugar was coming. Gone were the "good old days" of shakes and cold sweats. Now, mental confusion was the first noticeable sign that my blood sugar was dropping. And sometimes, it was too late for me to handle it on my own.

Thank God for my wife, Debbie. She's one of those rare people who knows just when to let me do my own thing and when to get involved. I met her in college and knew I would marry her after our first Valentine's Day together. She learned a few things about diabetes and went out of her way to prepare a huge heart-shaped box filled with popcorn and cashew nuts. You know what they say . . . The way to a man's heart is through his pancreas.

Debbie and I left St. Louis and moved to Chicago after we both graduated. While in Chicago, I met with a few more endocrinologists and other specialists about my diabetes. By this time, I was growing more and more frustrated with the constant swings between highs and lows. Nobody had any answers—just the same old rhetoric about "This is what your insulin is doing; you just need to adjust to it."

Then I had the most severe low blood sugar of my life. It came in the middle of the night after I had been playing full-court basketball earlier in the evening. According to Debbie, I was pale and completely unresponsive. My limbs jerked uncontrollably. She called for paramedics, and according to the reports, I fought them off pretty well while they tried to put an IV into my arm. When I finally regained consciousness, Debbie was standing next to me with an exhausted, worried look on her face. I looked to the side and saw tubes coming out of my arm. I also saw blood. My blood. On the pillow. On the sheets. On the floor. Everywhere.

That experience really shook me up. I found a guy at a nearby diabetes clinic who specialized in exercise. He gave me some suggestions about self-adjusting my long-acting insulin and eating extra food to prevent the nighttime lows after exercise, but he emphasized that my doctor would have to approve any such changes. It was the first time anyone had introduced the concept of self-adjusting my own doses. Why hadn't my doctor told me about this? And why in the world would I need his *approval* to make these kinds of changes?

That exercise physiologist opened my eyes to more than just a few minor dosage changes. He set me on an entirely new career path. I liked his approach so much that I decided to become an exercise physiologist for people with diabetes. So what if there were no full-time jobs for exercise physiologists at diabetes centers? I loved to exercise. I had diabetes. And I was on a mission to put the two together and help as many people as possible. So I went back to school, earned my master's degree in exercise physiology, and landed a position with the Joslin Diabetes Center's affiliate office in Philadelphia.

Being a New York/New Jersey native, Philadelphia seemed close enough to home—and it had its own NBA and NFL franchises (I don't think I could live in a city that did not have them). So we packed up and moved to Philly, where I became the Joslin Center's full-time exercise physiologist. I have to admit—my office was really cool. It had weights, treadmills, bikes, video equipment, and a great view of the sports complex in south Philly. The only thing better than my office was the team I worked with. The doctors, nurses, and dietitians were heavily into the concept of flexible insulin dosing and self-adjustment. I cross-trained with them at every opportunity and absorbed as much as I could about the many facets and components of diabetes care.

Perhaps the biggest breakthrough in terms of my own self-care was my decision in 1994 to try the insulin pump. Nobody at our center had used one, but there was mounting interest on the part of patients to have an insulin pump program. So I decided to be the guinea pig.

I'll never forget how nervous I was the day I got hooked up to that little gray box. There were about twenty doctors, nurses, and administrators watching my every move. Luckily, I had a super-nice trainer named Bob who coached me through the whole programming and infusion set change process. My first infusion set was a bent needle (the needle actually stayed in all the time). Soon, a flexible tube infusion set became available, followed by a set that could be disconnected and reconnected easily. Before that, you had to stay connected to the pump *all the time*—during showers, sports, even sex.

The pump's adjustable basal insulin patterns and mealtime bolusing feature really helped to stabilize my blood sugar levels. For the first time in almost 10 years, I could sleep past 8 a.m. without having my blood sugar skyrocket. I could delay my lunch without bottoming out. And best of all, I could work out to my heart's content without going low in the middle of the night. In fact, I haven't had a single severe low blood sugar since I started on the pump 10 years ago.

Along with pump therapy came a whole new approach to dietary management: carb counting. By counting the grams of carbohydrate in my meals and snacks, I can now eat what I choose as long as I match it with the correct dose of fast-acting insulin.

Speaking of insulin, the introduction of **insulin analogs** (lispro and aspart) in the late 1990s has had a tremendous impact on my diabetes management. Unlike Regular insulin, which takes 30 minutes to start working, 2 to 3 hours to peak and 5 to 6 hours to fade, the rapid-acting analogs peak in about an hour and only last 3 to 4 hours. They do the job and then get out of the way. Gone are my readings of over 300 right after eating. I can also be more spontaneous and flexible in terms of what I eat and when.

Of course, there have been a few other improvements along the way. My blood glucose meter now takes less than 1 microliter of blood and performs the test in 5 seconds. The old "Guillotine" has been replaced by an adjustable lancing pen with lancets that are micro-thin. I can barely feel the finger pricks anymore. If I choose, I can even take a reading from my arm or leg. I can do a Hemoglobin A1c in 4 minutes with a machine that I have in my office, and everything—from my pump to my meters to my carb counting book—is downloadable. Heck, my latest insulin pump can practically do my taxes for me!

Technology aside, the thing that has made the greatest difference in my life with diabetes is learning how to match my insulin to my needs. No more molding my life to fit my insulin program. Now, I shape the insulin program to fit my life.

As proud as I am of what we have accomplished in diabetes management, I can't help but recall how proud my original endocrinologist was with the state of things back in 1985. Twenty years from now, I'll probably look back to today and think, "Man, that was really archaic."

God, I hope so.

Why Manage?

Diabetes can be a dangerous and deadly illness—*if you let it*. Millions of people have had their lives shortened and seen the quality of their lives suffer, due to poorly managed diabetes.

There are countless examples of people with diabetes who have excelled in all aspects of life: professional athletes such as Jonathan Hayes (football), Catfish Hunter (baseball), Bobby Clarke (hockey), Chris Dudley (basketball), Bill Talbert (tennis), Michelle McGann (golf), Kris Freeman (skiing), and Gary Hall (swimming); entertainers such as Mary Tyler Moore (*The Dick Van Dyke* and *Mary Tyler Moore* shows), Jean Smart (*Designing Women*), and Zippora Karz (the New York City Ballet). Pioneers Bill Davidson (co-founder of Harley Davidson), Thomas Edison (inventor), Ernest Hemingway (author), and even Miss America 1999, Nicole Johnson.

Unfortunately, this group represents the minority of people with diabetes. More typical is my wife's grandmother, who lost her legs, her eyesight, and eventually her life to poor control of her diabetes.

Quality Diabetes Management: Long-Term Benefits

Have you ever spilled a sweet drink? Makes quite a sticky mess. Excess sugar in the bloodstream causes a sticky mess as well. Sugar sticks to proteins and cells in the blood, keeping them from performing their normal functions. It can also damage the smooth inner lining of blood vessels, making them susceptible to a variety of problems, from leaking to hardening to thickening and eventual clogging.

The damage caused by elevated blood sugar levels can begin within a few years of diagnosis. For those with type 2 diabetes, damage may already exist at the time of diagnosis, since the disease may have been present for many years. Diabetes is the fifth leading cause of death in the United States. It is the leading cause of blindness and new cases of kidney failure. It impairs circulation in the extremities, which limits the body's ability to fight infection. It damages nerve fibers that signal to us when a problem is present—further exposing us to injury and infection. As a result, diabetes contributes to more than 60,000 foot and leg amputations annually in the United States.

Diabetes is the most common cause of erectile dysfunction (impotency) in men, affecting 50–60% of all men with diabetes over age 50. It can also cause vaginal dryness and reduced sexual arousal. Diabetic nerve diseases cause a variety of digestive, thermoregulatory, urinary, and cardiovascular ailments. Heart disease and stroke are two to four times more common—and substantially more deadly—in people with diabetes. Poor diabetes management accelerates periodontal (gum) disease, resulting in oral infections and premature tooth loss for thousands of people. Because sugar tends to stick to the collagen surrounding tendons and ligaments, poorly controlled diabetes is linked to limited joint mobility syndromes such as frozen shoulder and trigger fingers.

Elevated blood sugar levels during pregnancy contribute to a variety of birth defects; the risk of miscarriage is four times greater for women with diabetes.

Overall, the annual health care cost for a person with diabetes exceeds $13,000 per year, compared to just over $2,500 for a person without diabetes. In 2002, treating diabetes and its complications in the United States cost more than $90 *billion*. Add nearly $40 billion in indirect costs resulting from disability and lost productivity, and the total annual cost of diabetes in the United States exceeds $130 billion.

Even though most diabetic complications appear several years after diagnosis, minor damage can begin within the first few years. Two major studies: The Diabetes Control and Complications Trial (DCCT–United States) and the United Kingdom Prospective Diabetes Study (UKPDS) confirmed that intense blood sugar control can dramatically reduce the risk for long-term diabetic complications.

In the DCCT, conducted from 1983 to 1993, more than 1,400 people with type 1 diabetes and mild (if any) existing complications were randomly assigned to either an intensive therapy group (three or more injections daily or use of an insulin pump; blood sugar testing four or more times daily; insulin dosage adjustment for diet/exercise), or a conventional therapy group (one or two fixed doses of insulin and one or two blood sugar tests daily). The participants were followed for an average of 6 years. The intensive therapy group had an average HbA1c of just over 7% (average blood sugar 150–160 mg/dl or 8.3–8.9 mmol), whereas the conventional therapy group was over 9% (average blood sugar 210–220 mg/dl, or 11.7–12.2 mmol). Intensive therapy reduced the risk of retinopathy (eye disease) by 76%, nephropathy (kidney disease) by 54%, and neuropathy (nerve disease) by 60%. The UKPDS produced similar results for people with type 2 diabetes.

> The DCCT and UKPDS research studies proved that intensive blood sugar control dramatically reduces the chances of developing long-term diabetic complications.

The math is quite simple. Every 1-point reduction in HbA1c corresponds with about a 30% reduction in your risk of developing complications. Amazing! If you lower your HbA1c from 10 to 9, you reduce your risk by 30%. Go from 9 to 8, another 30% reduction. Amazing! It's like getting a clearance discount on an item that is already on sale!

Of course, nothing is guaranteed. I've seen plenty of people with A1c's in the 6s and 7s who developed complications, and some in the 9s and 10s who never developed a problem. But the simple fact is this: Getting and keeping your A1c down puts the odds tremendously in your favor. With so many things beyond our control, it makes sense to do this one important thing to help ensure a healthy future.

Another long-term benefit of good blood sugar control is optimal growth. For children and adolescents, optimizing blood sugar levels will result in enhanced muscle and bone development. Elevated blood sugars typically reflect a deficiency of insulin, which is needed to fuel growing body tissues. Case in point: A high school basketball phenom, projected to be approximately 6'4" by the time he graduated, topped off at only 5'11" by the end of his senior year. The reason: During his junior and senior years, he all but ignored his diabetes, with his A1c climbing from 8% to over 14%. He grew only 1 inch during those 2 critical years and likely will never be more than 6 feet tall. Adequate insulin will help ensure that you reach your maximal height and muscle development.

Quality Diabetes Management: Short-Term Benefits

Immediate gratification—two words that motivate us like nothing else. If the thought of possibly preventing health problems several years from now fails to get you excited about controlling your blood sugars, perhaps these two words will.

Effective management of diabetes produces a number of important, immediate benefits:

Enhanced physical performance:
Improved blood glucose control will boost your strength, flexibility, stamina, speed, and overall energy level. Your reaction times will be quicker and you will recover from injuries more rapidly. Many of my patients have tracked their performance in a variety of sports (basketball, hockey, sprinting, swimming, lacrosse, tennis, etc.) and have consistently performed best when the blood sugars are well controlled. One young man's first MVP trophy coincided with the first time he managed to keep his blood sugar in the 100s (5.5–11

mmol) throughout a tournament. High blood sugar (hyper-glycemia) tends to produce dehydration, impair visual acuity, and slow reflexes. Muscle loss and cramping are also common side effects of hyperglycemia. Low blood sugars result in insufficient fuel for working muscles and may impair the brain's ability to coordinate movements. You're likely to see improved performance in everyday activities as well as athletics when your blood sugars are near normal.

Enhanced Intellectual Performance:

Proper blood sugar regulation will improve your ability to focus, memorize, and perform complex tasks. With hypoglycemia (low blood sugar), the brain is deprived of sufficient fuel to function properly. Repeated bouts of severe hypoglycemia can result in learning deficits. High blood sugars, on the other hand, tend to cause "sluggishness." The increased mental energy resulting from quality blood sugar control should yield positive results at work as well as school.

Enhanced Social/Coping Skills:

It didn't take my wife long to realize that my moods are affected by my blood sugar levels. For most people, low blood sugars cause a variety of unusual behaviors. High blood sugars impair our ability to deal with stress and interact effectively with other people. Irritability seems to increase with high blood sugars. Keeping your diabetes in check might just allow you to enhance your social standing and find simple solutions to many of your daily challenges.

Better Sleep:

Perhaps the only thing worse than a low blood sugar waking you up in the middle of the night is a full bladder causing you to toss and turn until, finally, you dash to the bathroom for a good 2-minute sugar-induced pee. Keeping your nighttime blood sugars under good control will allow you to get some well-deserved rest.

Fewer Infections:

High blood sugars create a virtual breeding ground for viruses and bacteria. Improving your blood sugar control should result in fewer and less severe infections—including vaginal yeast infections, skin infections, urinary tract infections, upper respiratory infections, and common colds.

Healthier Skin:

Another side effect of chronically high blood sugar is dry skin and an increased tendency towards acne. Maintaining normal blood sugar levels helps to keep skin moist and provides less fuel for bacteria-causing blemishes.

2

The Evolution
of Diabetes Care

LET ME START OUT by saying that I am *not* a history buff. Back
in school, I dreaded history class more than those greasy fish
sticks in the cafeteria. Perhaps it was because I had a hard time
applying all those names, dates, and events to my current life
situation. Of course, back then, my life situation consisted mostly
of sports, girls, fast food, and rock and roll—not necessarily in
that order.

Today, diabetes is a big part of my daily life, just as it is a big
part of yours. Whether you are new to diabetes or have been "pan-
creatically challenged" for many years, you can learn some valuable lessons from the evolution of diabetes care. It helps us to
understand what got us to this point and take advantage of what
is currently available. Most importantly, it lays the groundwork
for our future endeavors. After all, most great discoveries and
products of creativity are merely slight improvements over what
currently exists.

So let's take a look at how far we have come in the treatment of
diabetes. And, if history holds true (as it almost always does), we
can look forward to even greater improvements.

In the Beginning . . .

The first known case of diabetes was noted in the Ebers Papyrus, a document dating back to 1552 BC: Third Dynasty Egyptian physician Hesy-Ra described a patient whose primary symptom was incessant urination.

Sixteen hundred years later, in the first century AD, Greek physician Arateus described a mysterious illness that involved ". . . the melting down of flesh and limbs into urine. The patients never stop making water, but the flow is incessant, as if from the opening of aqueducts." Arateus coined the term "diabetes" from the Greek word meaning "siphon" or "pass through." Several years later, another Greek physician, Galen, came to the conclusion that diabetes must be a disease of the kidneys.

In 300 AD, Indian and Chinese scholars observed that the urine of people with diabetes was remarkably sweet. For the next 1,200 years, diabetes was commonly diagnosed by "water tasters" who drank the urine of those suspected of having diabetes. Another way to diagnose diabetes was to pour urine near an anthill. If the ants were attracted to the urine, it meant that the urine contained sugar. (I'm sure the "water tasters" appreciated this approach to diagnosis.) "Mellitus," the Latin word for honey, was later added to "diabetes" by Roman scientists.

Little progress was made until the 1600s, when English physician Matthew Dobson developed a method to extract sugar from both the blood and urine of people with diabetes. A French chemist, Chevreul, determined that the sugar in the blood and in the urine were both glucose. Thus the link between blood sugar and diabetes was established.

A century later, John Rollo demonstrated that the level of sugar in the urine corresponded to the types and amount of food eaten. Diets rich in breads, grains, and fruits tended to increase the amount of sugar excreted; diets consisting mainly of meats tended to decrease it. Rollo theorized that the diseased organ in diabetes was the stomach, which he thought overproduced sugar from plant matter. However, the "sick stomach" theory did not last long.

English physician Thomas Cawley, while performing an autopsy on a patient with diabetes, noticed that the pancreas of a diabetic man seemed different than that of a healthy person. From that point on, the pancreas became the locus of research in diabetes.

In the mid-1800s, a German medical student named Paul Langerhans discovered clusters of cells in the pancreas that resembled islands in the sea. Although he could not describe their function, the cells became known as the **Islets of Langerhans**. In 1889, two Austrian scientists named Minkowski and Mering bickered about whether a dog could survive without a pancreas. They removed the pancreas and observed that the previously housebroken animal urinated profusely. Flies swarmed around the sweet urine. Lucky for Minkowski, the first chemical tests to measure sugar in urine (no more "water tasting"!) were being developed. Minkowski tested the urine and found that it contained large amounts of glucose. He also noted that the dogs ". . . threw themselves at any time upon the food which was offered to them, even when they had, only a short time before, been amply fed, and all the time they looked around for every drop of water they could get a hold of."

The First Treatments

By the late 1800s, a variety of treatments were being tested for diabetes mellitus. Theorizing about the rapid loss of sugar through the urine, a French physician (Priorry) advised his patients to eat as much sugar as possible, to replace what was being lost. Another French physician, Bouchardat, noticed that urine sugar levels of patients dropped with the rationing of food during the Franco-Prussian War. He formulated the idea of individualized, restrictive diets for his diabetes patients. Catoni, an Italian diabetes specialist, actually placed his patients under lock and key, to force them to follow their prescribed low-calorie diet.

In the early 1900s, a number of other "fad" treatments arose, including the "oatmeal cure," the all-milk diet, the rice diet, potato therapy, opium treatment, and bloodletting. Frederick Allen of the United States published his dietary recommendations for diabetes, which emphasized an extremely low-calorie diet. Although most patients' symptoms improved, many died from malnourishment. The average life expectancy for a newly diagnosed patient was 1 to 4 years.

German scientist Georg Zuelzer developed the first injectable pancreatic extract to block the flow of sugar into the urine. The extract was administered to de-pancreatized dogs. The resulting seizures (likely due to hypoglycemia) were thought to be toxic effects, and the experiments were suspended.

Then came the "Roaring Twenties." Frederick Banting and his assistant, Charles Best, at the University of Toronto, used an innovative technique for isolating the secretions from the Islets of Langerhans. An extract taken from a fetal calf cured the diabetes of dogs whose pancreases had been removed. It was then tried on Leonard Thompson, a 14-year-old boy who was dying from diabetes. Thompson showed little improvement.

A biochemist, J. B. Collip, purified Banting and Best's extract, and the experiment was repeated 12 days later. This time, Thompson began to gain weight; he went on to live another 15 years, with regular injections. A Toronto physician with severe diabetes, Joe Gilchrist, also received the extract—as did an American, James Havens. Soon, a multitude of near-death patients showed up at Banting and Best's doorstep. For the first time, diabetes was transformed from a slow death sentence to a treatable chronic disease. Banting was awarded the Nobel Prize in Medicine, and Eli Lilly and Company agreed to engage in the bulk production of the magical extract known as "insulin."

"Real" Treatment Begins

Below are the decade-by-decade highlights in the management of diabetes since the discovery of insulin.

1920s

Initially, mass-produced insulin was extracted from the pancreases of cattle and pigs. Its high level of impurity (more than 50,000 parts per million) caused frequent skin infections and inconsistent action. It had a relatively short duration of activity, with a peak at approximately 3 hours and a 6-hour duration. As a result, patients had to inject their insulin (a brownish extract) every 6 to 8 hours, using large glass syringes. Dosing was based on the appearance of symptoms: Increase the dosage if urination increased; decrease the dosage if hypoglycemic symptoms (or seizures) appeared.

1930s

Researchers developed a long-acting insulin by combining regular insulin with protamine, a protein found in fish sperm. With a duration of action of 36 hours, users of protamine-zinc insulin (PZI) had to take an injection every day and a half. This odd schedule caused confusion and dosing lapses/overlaps for many patients. Doses were adjusted based on symptoms.

1940s

A statistical connection was found between diabetes and kidney and eye diseases. The first standardized insulin syringe was developed to help make dosing more uniform. It was a glass syringe with a reusable steel needle that needed to be boiled between uses to assure sterility (see Figure 2-1). The needle was reused until it became too dull to puncture the skin. Most patients received one insulin injection daily. Dietary plans focused on complete avoidance of sugary foods but ample consumption of other "normal" foods, as reduced rates of infection were observed in well-fed (vs. undernourished) individuals. The average life expectancy for a person with diabetes was about 30 years.

1950s

The full extent of long-term diabetic **complications** became apparent as many patients lived long enough with diabetes to experience

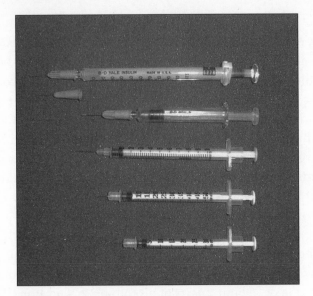

Figure 2-1: Early insulin syringes have undergone a major transformation over the past 70+ years.

blindness, kidney failure, heart disease, amputations, and a variety of nerve disorders. An official distinction was made between type 1 and type 2 diabetes. Eliot Joslin spoke out on the value of tight blood sugar control, using many of his patients as examples. Intermediate-acting insulins (NPH and Lente) were developed. Their duration of action allowed patients the convenience of once-daily injections. Exercise was recognized as a helpful way to "burn up extra glucose." Urine testing for glucose was the norm: Simply take a test tube of water, add four drops of urine, then drop in a magical tablet to make it fizz. Watch the color changes to determine whether your blood sugar level was normal, high, very high, or ridiculously high several hours ago (urine glucose levels lag several hours behind blood glucose levels). A messy process, but it still beat the old "water tasting" routine from ancient times!

1960s

The purity of insulin improved considerably, to approximately 20,000 impure parts per million. Blood glucose levels were measured routinely during visits to the doctor's office. Insulin was sold in three concentrations: U-40, U-80, and U-100 (the higher the number, the "purer" and more concentrated the insulin). The insulin concentration had to be matched to syringes with the same concentration markings. One or two injections of NPH and Regular insulin daily were the norm. Ultralente offered another option for long-acting insulin. "Tes-Tape" replaced the test tube method for measuring urine glucose levels. Simply pee on the tape; if it turns yellow, the blood glucose level several hours earlier was normal. Black means it was high. Shades of gray are up to the user's discretion.

The "diabetic exchange diet" also made its debut. Developed to give patients multiple food options and distribute fat, protein, and carbohydrate intake evenly throughout the day, it forced many people into very rigid, strict meal plans. It was also complex and required intense attention to portion measurement. Sweets were still considered "taboo" in the diabetic's diet.

1970s

The first blood glucose meters and insulin pumps were developed. These devices were bulky and generally unreliable (see Figure 2-2). The meters utilized crude photometrics (color change on a test strip) to measure glucose concentrations of the blood. The first insulin pumps infused a single rate of basal insulin throughout the day and whole-unit doses at meals. They were plagued by clogs and insulin stability problems, resulting in frequent episodes of ketoacidosis. Short-acting (Regular, Semi-lente), intermediate-acting (NPH, Lente, Globin), and long-acting (Ultralente, Protamine Zinc) insulins were all in use. U-40 and U-80 insulin and syringes were phased out in favor of the standard U-100 versions. Disposable syringes became available. The standard of care called for two injections per day of intermediate- and long-acting insulin. By providing basal insulin throughout the day and larger doses at meals, this program was an improvement over previous regimens but provided little flexibility for the patient.

1980s

Human insulin, synthesized through recombinant DNA technology,

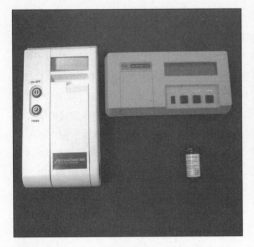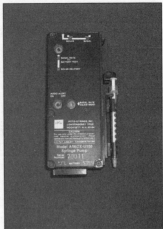

Figure 2-2: Early meters and pump

became available. This type of insulin caused fewer allergic reactions and less **autoimmunity** than animal-derived insulin. And because it was produced in a laboratory, the supply of insulin became virtually limitless. Insulin pens were developed, enabling more discrete and accurate injections. Blood glucose meters became more streamlined and accurate. Insulin pumps, while still not widely popular, became safer and more portable. Needle-less "jet" injectors were introduced. The first computer programs became available for analyzing data from blood glucose meters. The Hemoglobin A1c test was developed, allowing assessment of long-term blood glucose control. Carbohydrate gram counting and carb exchanges/choices became accepted methods for balancing food intake against insulin doses. Two or three injections daily was the standard of care.

1990s

Results of the **DCCT** were reported and published; treatment focused on tighter control of blood glucose levels. Insulin pumps grew in popularity, as advanced programming features and soft-tube/disconnectable infusion sets were developed. Blood glucose meters became much smaller, faster, and more precise. The first insulin analog, lispro, came into use. With its rapid absorption and short, consistent action, it became the insulin of choice for use at mealtimes. Internet-based diabetes management programs and patient-centered chat rooms helped to spread the word about intensive diabetes therapy. Carbohydrate gram counting increased in popularity; patients were more routinely taught to self-adjust insulin based on food, activity, and blood glucose levels. "Short-needle," ultra-thin syringes and lancets made insulin administration and blood glucose testing significantly more comfortable.

2000 to Today

Continuous glucose monitoring, though still somewhat rudimentary, has become available to the public by way of the GlucoWatch Biographer (Cygnus Corporation) and Continuous Glucose Monitoring System (Medtronic/MiniMed). Alternate-site blood glucose meters, which permit testing at sites other than the fingertips, have reached the forefront. At-home and mail-order HbA1c testing has become available. The first peakless "basal" insulins (Lantus and Detemir) have been developed. Several new companies with various computerized innovations have entered the insulin pump market, and insulin pump use is increasing at a rapid rate, particularly among children and seniors. Multiple daily injections (background insulin plus fast-acting insulin taken at mealtimes) are becoming more common. Handheld computers can be used to manage diabetes self-care records and offer insight for achieving better control.

Looking Ahead

Manufacturers are currently developing alternative methods for administering insulin, including inhalers, nasal devices, pills, and skin patches. However, these types of devices do little to help us think more like a pancreas; they only offer a more convenient and (perhaps) pain-free method for administering insulin.

Research is underway to determine the precise effects of fat, protein, and various vitamin/mineral supplements on blood sugar regulation. The role of the glycemic index (the rate at which different foods digest and convert into blood sugar) is being studied as it applies to diabetes management. Soon we may have sophisticated algorithms for matching insulin to our diets based on the specific components of the food.

The importance of after-meal (postprandial) blood glucose control has gained recognition in recent years. Industry leaders are working to develop lifestyle and medical approaches to help minimize postprandial hyperglycemia.

Two methods for achieving optimal, automatic blood glucose regulation are in development. One involves the transplantation of insulin-producing islet cells. Although this method has been proven effective for achieving near-perfect blood glucose control in hundreds of patients worldwide, it is hindered by the limited number of available islet cells and the need for immunosuppressant drugs. Although nonsteroidal, these drugs have a tendency to produce a number of negative side effects.

The second major effort involves the development of "closed-loop" technology: linking a continuous glucose sensor with an insulin pump. Essentially, the sensor reads the blood sugar and tells the pump when to start and stop releasing insulin. Some research and development companies are working on systems that would be implanted inside the body (like an artificial pancreas); others are taking external body surface meters and pumps and working to make them communicate with each other.

Despite these and other recent innovations, only a small percentage of people with diabetes manages to achieve the kind of blood sugar control recommended by medical experts. Diabetes remains a leading cause of blindness, kidney failure, heart disease, stroke, limb amputation, and nerve disease. The acute (short-term) complications of diabetes, such as severe hypoglycemia and ketoacidosis, result in countless accidents and billions of dollars in lost earnings due to short-term disability. The average life expectancy of a person with diabetes remains 13 years less than that of a person without diabetes.

As history has shown time and time again, technology alone does not drive us toward success. It is how we *apply* technology that makes the difference. It takes an informed, motivated person, utilizing technology to the fullest, to manage diabetes effectively. This will be the focus of the remainder of the book.

3

Mastering the Basics

MANAGING YOUR DIABETES IS like building a home. Before you can even think about fancy fixtures and color patterns, you must have a solid foundation. Prior to jumping into the intricacies of blood glucose regulation, let's take a few moments to get acquainted (or reacquainted) with some diabetes fundamentals. Even if you think you know all the basics, keep in mind that our knowledge of diabetes is constantly expanding. Here's your chance to get caught up on all the latest facts.

Type 1 Versus Type 2

If you ask an endocrinologist to describe the different forms of diabetes, you'd better have some snacks handy because you're in for a long discussion. In recent years, many new forms of diabetes have been designated. Many are combinations of type 1 and type 2, while others have pregnancy as a component.

I prefer to put diabetes into two major classes: the kind caused by beta cell destruction (type 1), and the kind caused by insulin resistance (type 2). All people with type 1 diabetes need to take insulin to survive. Many people with type 2 diabetes also take insulin, but mainly as a tool for achieving effective blood sugar control.

Type 1 and type 2 diabetes both cause blood sugar levels to be too high. Both can result in **hypoglycemia** (low blood sugar) when insulin or insulin-increasing medications (sulfonylureas or meglitinides) are used in the treatment. Both require careful ongoing management. And both can cause a wide range of health problems (complications). However, the similarities stop there. From a physiological standpoint, type 1 and type 2 are as different as chocolate and vanilla. First, let's look at the chocolate, er . . . type 1 diabetes.

Type 1 diabetes involves a lack of insulin production from the pancreas, usually due to destruction of insulin-producing cells by the body's own immune system.

Type 1 diabetes, for lack of a better definition, refers to a lack of internal insulin production. Insulin comes from the pancreas, an organ just below the stomach. There are groups of cells in the pancreas called "islet" cells, and within the islets are "beta" cells. Beta cells constantly measure blood sugar levels and produce insulin as needed, to keep the blood sugar level within a normal range.

In type 1 diabetes, the beta cells are destroyed either by trauma (accidents, cancer, severe pancreatitis) or, more commonly, by the body's own immune system, rendering the pancreas unable to produce any insulin. Normally, the immune system only attacks things that are foreign to your own body. In an autoimmune disease such as diabetes, the immune system fails to recognize something as part of your body and attacks it. In the case of type 1 diabetes, the islet cells are attacked and destroyed over a period of months or years. As a result, the blood sugar level goes up and the body's cells are deprived of the sugar they need to burn for energy.

Presently, there are approximately one million people in the United States with type 1 diabetes, with 20,000 to 30,000 new diagnoses made every year. Type 1 diabetes is usually diagnosed during childhood and adolescence, but it can also appear during adulthood. The incidence of type 1 diabetes is increasing at a steady rate as adults with type 1 diabetes are living longer and having more children than ever before.

Just before diagnosis, a person with type 1 diabetes will likely have very high blood sugar levels and will be producing little or no insulin. Very high blood sugar levels cause excessive urination as the kidneys eliminate some of the sugar through the urine. In essence, you will be urinating away almost everything you eat. Losing all those fluids will make you very thirsty. And since you will be unable to get sugar into your cells, your energy level will be low and you will have to resort to fat as your only source of energy. Consequently, rapid weight loss can occur.

Soon after diagnosis with type 1 diabetes, insulin treatment begins. This initial treatment can provide a recovery period for any remaining beta cells. As a result, these remaining cells may be able to produce enough insulin to keep blood sugar levels relatively stable for a period of weeks, months, or even years. We refer to this as the "**honeymoon phase**" (or, using married life as an analogy, I like to call it "the calm before the storm"). Eventually, beta cell function ceases and insulin requirements increase. Without insulin, a person with type 1 diabetes will eventually fall into a coma and die. This is the reason type 1 diabetes is also called "insulin-dependent" diabetes: You depend on insulin to live.

Of the 16 million Americans who have diabetes, approximately 15 million have type 2. Almost all people with type 2 diabetes still produce some of their own insulin. They may take insulin to keep the blood sugar under control, but insulin is usually not necessary for short-term survival.

Type 2 diabetes is a progressive disease. Initially, high blood sugars are caused by insulin resistance. Eventually insulin production falters, resulting in the need for more aggressive treatment.

Type 2 diabetes is caused by insulin resistance: a condition in which insulin's normal blood sugar–lowering action is inhibited. More insulin than usual is required to keep blood sugar levels under control. People with type 1 diabetes can also experience insulin resistance, but usually not to the same extent as people with type 2.

What causes insulin resistance? Typically, it is caused by a combination of genetic and lifestyle factors. Heredity plays a major role; having close relatives with type 2 diabetes greatly increases your risk. Certain ethnic groups, including Native Americans, African Americans, and Hispanics, are also at a high risk. Insulin resistance increases along with body size. Body fat, particularly around the abdomen, tends to interfere with insulin action. Men whose waist measurement (at navel level) is greater than 40" (102 cm), and women who are greater than 35" (88 cm) are considered to have abdominal obesity. Lack of exercise and a diet high in calories contribute to this problem, as does a stressful lifestyle. Pregnancy can cause insulin resistance, due to increases in weight and production of placental hormones that raise blood sugar levels.

Type 2 diabetes is a progressive illness. This does not mean that it is hip, cool, or modern. Type 2 diabetes is progressive because it starts small and grows worse over time. In the early stages, type 2 diabetes can often be controlled through exercise and a healthy diet. Over time, as the pancreas starts losing the ability to produce insulin, oral medications designed to improve insulin production or enhance its action may need to be added. Eventually, insulin may be added to offset the combination of low insulin production and insulin resistance. Approximately 40% of people diagnosed with type 2 diabetes currently take insulin.

To understand how this progression occurs, imagine that you are running an air conditioner to keep your house cool in the summer. Whenever the temperature goes up, the thermostat kicks the air conditioner on. However, something isn't quite right with your system. The freezer component has a leak, and the system is blowing air that is just cool, instead of cold. The temperature in the house remains slightly elevated all the time, causing the air conditioner to run most of the time. After a few days, you notice that the air coming out of the vent is lukewarm, and that the system is running nonstop. Know what happens to a machine that runs nonstop without any breaks? Yep—it breaks down. That is what happens to the pancreas. After being overworked for an extended period of time, it literally burns itself out. As production of insulin drops off, more potent forms of treatment are required to control blood sugar levels.

Treatment of type 2 diabetes begins with healthy lifestyle habits: a sensible diet, regular exercise, stress management, and sound preventive health care. These approaches are critical for the prevention of long-term complications, achievement of a healthy body weight, and maintenance of a high quality of life. They are also the cornerstones of effective blood glucose management. Insulin therapy is essential to blood glucose regulation in all people with type 1 diabetes and those with type 2 diabetes whose disease is at an advanced stage. The bottom line: Regardless of which type of diabetes you have, it is very important to live a healthy lifestyle and control your blood sugar levels.

The Science Behind Blood Sugar Regulation

Blood sugar comes from two sources: internal and external. Internal sources are sugars that are stored up in the liver and, to a lesser extent, the muscles. External sources are the food we eat—mainly carbohydrates. Internal and external sugar is converted into a specific type of sugar called **glucose** for circulation in the bloodstream.

Insulin is necessary to get the glucose out of the bloodstream and into the body's cells so that it can be burned for energy. Glucose is the preferred energy source for most cells of the body. Some cells, such as brain cells, will only burn glucose for energy. Thus, it is very important to have a steady supply of glucose available in the bloodstream.

Besides helping get sugar out of the bloodstream and into the body's cells, insulin has another job: blocking the release of sugar from the liver and muscles. Instead, insulin packs sugar into the liver for use at another time.

When a person without diabetes has not eaten for a while, the blood sugar level can come down. This can occur between meals, during sleep, and especially during exercise. When the blood sugar begins to drop, the pancreas decreases its production of insulin and increases its production of a second hormone: **glucagon**. Not only does this reduce the amount of sugar being taken out of the bloodstream, it also forces the liver to release some of its stored-up sugar. As a result, blood sugar levels don't go too low.

In a way, the pancreas acts like the thermostat that keeps your house comfy-cozy. When the temperature goes up, the thermostat kicks on the fan. When the temperature goes down, the thermostat kicks on the heat. That way, the temperature stays within a comfortable range.

In you body, when the blood sugar level begins to rise, the pancreas secretes extra insulin, which brings the blood sugar level down. When the blood sugar level falls, the pancreas eases back on insulin production and begins producing glucagon, which brings the blood sugar back up. This system helps keep the blood sugar within a range that is comfy-cozy for your body: approximately 60 to 110 (3.3–6.1 mmol).

Factors that Affect Blood Sugars

Here is where the science becomes something of an art. Different things affect different people differently under different circumstances.

A major part of blood sugar management involves integrating all the factors that affect your blood sugar levels and trying to make them all balance out. If the factors that raise your blood sugar are equal to the factors that lower it, your blood sugar level should remain fairly steady.

There are a few major factors that affect our blood sugars on a regular basis, and a number of minor factors that occur on special occassions (see Figure 3-1). Let's start with the major factors.

Major Factors Affecting Blood Sugar

<u>Raise Blood Sugar</u>	<u>Lower Blood Sugar</u>
⇑ Food ⇑	⇓ Physical Activity ⇓
⇑ Stress ⇑	⇓ Insulin ⇓
⇑ Illness ⇑	⇓ Oral Diabetes Medication ⇓

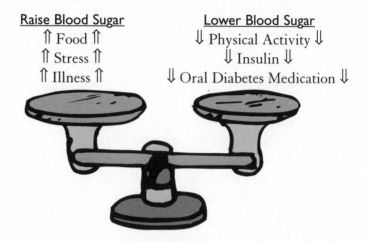

Factor 1: Insulin

Insulin lowers blood sugar. Plain and simple. However, the exact action of insulin varies depending on factors such as the type of insulin, rate of absorption from below the skin, the source of the insulin, and the body's sensitivity to the insulin.

Insulin is measured in units. A unit of insulin will lower the blood sugar the same amount, no matter what kind of insulin you use. A unit of fast-acting insulin will lower your blood sugar the same as a unit of long-acting insulin; it just does so in a shorter period of time. One exception is a new basal insulin called Detemir, which has a potency that is approximately 75% less than that of all other insulins.

Another exception occurs when the insulin concentration varies. Worldwide, most insulin is standardized as "U-100." This means that there are 100 units of insulin in every cc (cubic centimeter) of fluid. In rare instances, diluted (U-50) or concentrated (U-400) insulin can be found. Some people choose to dilute their insulin to as little as U-10, to allow dosing in more precise increments with standard insulin syringes. For example, a child who is very sensitive to insulin may have his/her insulin diluted to U-10 by mixing 90 units of neutral diluent with 10 units of insulin. The resulting mixture would have 10% of the potency of normal U-100 insulin. One unit (as measured on an insulin syringe) would actually be equivalent to one-tenth of a unit of U-100 insulin.

A summary of insulin types is given below (see Table 3-1). Be aware that the precise action times can vary considerably from person to person.

Because insulin is injected (or infused, in the case of an insulin pump) into the fat below the skin, the exact onset, peak, and duration can vary depending on a number of factors.

Analog insulins are similar to human insulin, but with slight alterations so as to effectively control their onset, peak, and duration of action. The actions of insulin "analogs" (Humalog, Novolog, Lantus, Detemir) are not affected very much by injection sites, but older-generation insulins (Regular, NPH, Lente, Ultralente) can vary considerably.

In general, the action of the older-generation insulins is more rapid in body parts that have greater blood flow below the skin. Injecting the abdomen tends to produce the most rapid absorption, followed by the arms, then the legs, and finally the buttocks. When using non-analog insulins, keep your injection sites consistent. For example, always use the abdomen in the morning, thigh at dinner, and buttocks at bedtime.

Injecting a non-analog insulin into a body part that will be exercising may also accelerate the action of the insulin—particularly when the exercise is performed within an hour or two of the injection. This is due to the greatly enhanced blood flow in the area that is being used. For example, injecting into the thigh and then running may result in an earlier onset/peak and shorter duration of insulin action.

The source of the insulin can also affect its action. Many non-analog insulins are available as either human (identical to human insulin) or animal (identical to cow or pig) varieties. Human insulins tend to work somewhat faster than animal insulins. Because animal insulins tend to cause greater immune responses than human

Rapid-Acting Insulin Analog (*Humalog, Novolog*)
Starts: 5–15 min   Peaks: ¾–1½ hrs   Lasts: 3–4 hrs

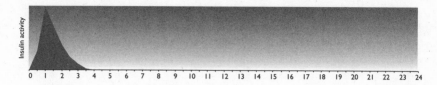

Short-Acting Insulin (*Regular*)
Starts: 15–30 min   Peaks: 2–3 hrs   Lasts: 4–6 hrs

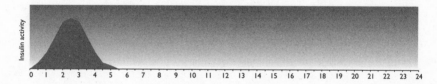

Intermediate-Acting Insulin (*NPH, Lente*)*
Starts: 1–2 hrs   Peaks: 4–8 hrs   Lasts: 12–18 hrs

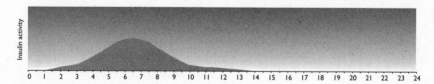

Long-Acting Insulin (*Ultralente*)*
Starts: 4–6 hrs   Peaks: 8–18 hrs   Lasts: 20–24 hrs

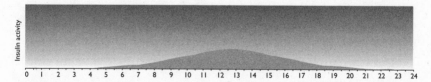

*Cloudy insulin mixtures must be rolled vigorously to ensure an even mixture and consistent concentration.

Table 3-1: Types of insulin and their actions

Basal Insulin Analog (*Lantus*)
Starts: 1–3 hrs   Peaks: none   Lasts: 20–24 hrs

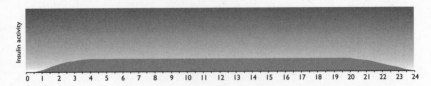

Basal Insulin Analog (*Detemir*)
Starts: 1–2 hrs   Peaks: none   Lasts: 12–16 hrs

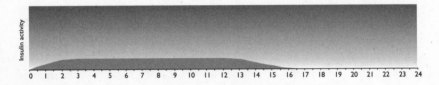

Table 3-1: Types of insulin and their actions (continued)

insulins, they are generally not recommended unless slower insulin action is absolutely necessary.

Insulin action can also be affected by a condition known as lipodystrophy. Repeated injections into the same small area of skin can cause the fat below the skin to either swell and harden (lipohypertrophy) or wear away (lipoatrophy). In either case, the absorption of insulin will be affected. For this reason, it is best to "rotate" your injection sites—move the site of needle penetration around over a large area of skin. If it helps, imagine that you have a monthly calendar printed on each of the body parts where you inject, and inject into the spot that corresponds with the day of the month.

Below are a few other notes to help ensure that your insulin is working as expected:

Storage: Unopened insulin vials/cartridges should be stored in a refrigerator (but not frozen). This will keep your insulin "fresh" until the expiration date. The butter compartment on the door might make an ideal home. Once a vial or cartridge is opened (i.e., the rubber stopper is punctured), it can be kept at room temperature for up to 1 month. Room-temperature insulin tends to form fewer bubbles in the syringe and is generally more comfortable to inject. Your insulin should be kept out of direct sunlight and away from heating devices. When ordering insulin through the mail, request that it be shipped in a thermally insulated package. When traveling, keep your insulin in a cushioned pouch and do *not* leave it in a car or bus for more than a few minutes. Do not use insulin that has an unusual appearance. If it has crystals on the surface, does not mix uniformly, has residue at the bottom even after mixing, or has an unusual color, it should be discarded.

Replacement: Insulin vials and cartridges should not be used for more than a month. When in use, contaminants and impurities find their way into your insulin and cause it to start losing potency. Every month, discard whatever you have left and start new vials/cartridges.

Mixing Technique: Most insulins (with the exception of Lantus) may be mixed with each other in a syringe immediately prior to injection (see Table 3-2). Because of its slight acidic property, Lantus should never be mixed with another insulin. To ensure that your insulin is not contaminated during the mixing process, be sure to draw up insulin in order from fastest- to slowest-acting. In other words, draw the clear (fast) insulin into your syringe before drawing in the cloudy (slow) insulin. If a tiny amount of fast-acting insulin gets into the vial of slow-acting insulin, it usually will not cause any harm. However, if slow-acting insulin gets into the vial of fast-acting insulin, it will contaminate the entire vial.

Proper Injection: Whether you use syringes, pens, or a pump, elimination of large air bubbles is important. Very small (soda-sized)

	Humalog	Novolog	Regular	NPH	Lente	Ultralente	Detemir	Lantus
Humalog	•	N/A	YES	YES	YES	YES	YES	NO
Novolog	N/A	•	YES	YES	YES	YES	YES	NO
Regular	YES	YES	•	YES	YES	YES	YES	NO
NPH	YES	YES	YES	•	NO	NO	NO	NO
Lente	YES	YES	YES	NO	•	YES	NO	NO
Ultralente	YES	YES	YES	NO	YES	•	NO	NO
Detemir	YES	YES	YES	NO	NO	NO	•	NO
Lantus	NO	NO	NO	NO	NO	NO	NO	•

Table 3-2: Okay to mix?

bubbles are not much of a concern, but larger bubbles will cause your insulin dose to be reduced significantly. As mentioned previously, room-temperature insulin that is rolled (rather than shaken) is less likely to form bubbles. Next, make sure that the insulin is injected at the proper depth. Select a needle that is the proper length for your body type, and pinch the skin when injecting/inserting. Release the pinch after injecting and, if using a pen, keep the needle in for 5 to 10 seconds, to ensure complete insulin delivery.

If the process of inserting the needle into the skin leaves you gasping for breath, a number of "injection aids" are available, including the Inject-Ease (Palco Labs), Automatic Injector (BD), Pen Mate for the insulin pen (Novo Nordisk), and the Sil-Serter, Sof-Serter, and Quick-Serter for pump infusion sets (Medtronic/MiniMed).

Factor 1A: Insulin/Medication Combinations
Many people with type 2 diabetes take oral medication along with their insulin. These medications work in a variety of ways, but all are designed to lower blood sugar levels. Table 3-3 reviews these.

Factor 2: Food
Whoever said that there is no such thing as a free lunch really knew what he was talking about.

Drug Class	Examples	Action
Sulfonylureas	Glucotrol, Micronase, Amaryl	Stimulate the pancreas to secrete more insulin throughout the day and night
Meglitinides	Prandin, Starlix	Stimulate the pancreas to secrete more insulin for a short period of time (after meals)
Alpha Glucosidase Inhibitors	Precose, Glyset	Slow the digestion/absorption of carbohydrates
Biguanides	Glucophage	Suppress the secretion of sugar by the liver
Thiazoladinediones	Actos, Avandia	Enhance the body's sensitivity to insulin

Table 3-3: Oral diabetes medications

Just about everything we eat (or drink) causes the blood sugar to rise, with one exception: water. In fact, staying well hydrated can actually lower blood sugar levels somewhat. Otherwise, it's all up from there.

The three major nutrients found in food are protein, fat, and carbohydrate. Protein's effect on blood sugar is minimal. Very little, if any, protein "converts" into glucose. However, large amounts of protein, such as large portions of beef, fish, poultry, and eggs, can have a "sparing" effect on glucose metabolism, resulting in a gradual rise in the blood sugar level.

Likewise, dietary fat's impact on blood sugar is usually of little significance. However, consumption of large amounts of fat can cause a prolonged rise in the blood sugar level. Exactly why this happens is not entirely clear. Some researchers believe that large amounts of fat in the bloodstream contribute to temporary insulin resistance. Others contend that a small portion of fat converts into glucose. Whatever the cause, high fat intake has a tendency to cause modest increases in blood sugar levels over the course of many hours.

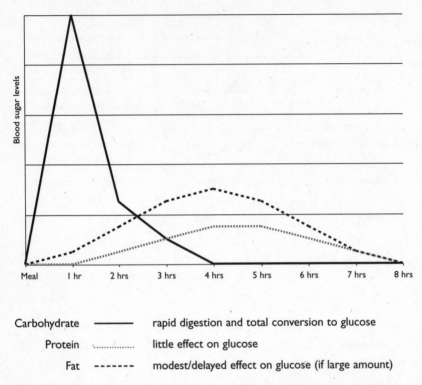

Carbohydrate	———	rapid digestion and total conversion to glucose
Protein	··················	little effect on glucose
Fat	- - - - - -	modest/delayed effect on glucose (if large amount)

Table 3-4: Nutrient Absorption: Timed effect on blood sugar levels

Carbohydrates are the nutrients that have the primary effect on blood sugar levels. Carbohydrates (or "carbs," for short) include simple sugars like glucose, sucrose (table sugar), fructose (fruit sugar), and lactose (milk sugar), as well as complex carbohydrates, better known as "starch." Think of simple sugars as individual railroad cars, and starch as a whole bunch of cars linked together to make a train. Most starches are composed of many glucose molecules linked together.

When you eat something that contains starch, the individual sugar molecules become unhooked from each other. This process takes place very quickly, beginning the moment food comes in contact with saliva. The individual glucose molecules start reaching the bloodstream within minutes.

Don't be overly concerned about the sugar content of a food. Be concerned about the total carbohydrate content.

From the standpoint of blood sugar control, it doesn't matter much whether the carbohydrates you eat are in the form of simple sugars or starches. Both will raise the blood sugar by the same amount. A cup of rice containing 45 grams of complex carbohydrates (starch) will raise the blood sugar just as much as a can of regular, sugar-sweetened soda that contains 45 grams of simple carbohydrates (sugar). And both will do it pretty fast.

*   *   *

Foods rich in sugar (simple carbohyrdates)	Foods rich in starch (complex carbohydrates)
Fruit	Potatoes
Fruit juice	Rice
Regular soda	Noodles/pasta
Candy	Cereal
Chocolate	Oatmeal
Cookies and cakes	Bread
Milk	Bagels
Ice cream	Crackers
Frozen yogurt	Tortillas
Table sugar	Pancakes
Honey	Beans
Syrup	Corn
Jelly	Salty snacks
	Beer

Table 3-5: Some foods rich in carbohydrates

Also, beware of "sugar-free" products. Having spent three years working in advertising, I can tell you that marketing people will do just about anything to get you to buy their products—even if it means bending the truth a little. "Sugar Free" can be put on a food label if the food does not contain sucrose (table sugar). However, a sugar-free food *can* contain complex carbohydrates, fructose (fruit sugar), and a variety of "sugar substitutes" such as sorbitol, xylitol, mannitol, lactitol, isomalt, and maltodextrin—all of which raise the blood sugar as much as ordinary sugar.

There are only a few artificial sweeteners that have little or no

> *"Sugar Free" simply means that a food contains no sucrose (table sugar). It can contain other sugars as well as complex carbohydrates.*

effect on blood sugar levels. These include saccharin, acesulfame K, sucralose (Splenda), and aspartame (NutraSweet); NutraSweet is found in many diet soft drinks, candies, yogurts, and other common foods. But be careful: Even if a product label says that it contains aspartame (or NutraSweet), it may also contain sugar substitutes that will raise your blood sugar level. *Always read the label* for the total carbohydrate content of a food before assuming that it is a "free food."

If you're used to using an exchange diet and assuming that foods like fat-free salad dressing and certain fresh vegetables don't count against your blood sugar, think again. Many fat-free foods use sugar or sugar substitutes to add flavor and texture, so check your labels. And even salad vegetables contain *some* carbohydrates. Remember, every carb (with the exception of **fiber**) counts toward your blood sugar!

Make it a priority to get good at counting the grams of carbohydrate

> *A major part of "thinking like a pancreas" involves matching insulin to carbohydrate intake.*

in your meals and snacks. More information on counting carbohydrates as well as helpful hints can be found in the next chapter.

Factor 3: Physical Activity

Physical activity is a potent tool for lowering blood sugar. It does this by burning up large amounts of sugar and improving the way insulin works—a process better known as "**insulin sensitivity**."

Imagine insulin as a key that opens doors to your cells, allowing sugar to ramble inside and get burned up for energy. Now, imagine that you temporarily lose your senses and decide to paint the entire outside of your home. Yourself. With no real painting skills per se. All of a sudden, your cells have a need for lots more energy. The few doors that exist on your muscle cells don't allow the sugar to get in fast enough. The solution, as you might have guessed, is for your body's cells to make more doors. And that's just what happens.

Suddenly, those insulin keys have more doors to open, and sugar is able to flow easily out of the bloodstream and into your cells. Now you have the energy you need to clean up the huge mess you created by dropping the paint can onto the roof of your car.

Unfortunately, nothing lasts forever. The extra doors built by the body's cells are only temporary. After being sedentary for a few hours, the doors get taken down and you start going back to the way things were before your activity level increased. In fact, extended periods of inactivity can reduce sensitivity to insulin, resulting in a state of **insulin resistance**. This, of course, is a major characteristic of type 2 diabetes.

What's that, you say? You've heard that blood sugar can go up during exercise? True, it can. But it is not the physical activity that causes it. Physical activity always improves insulin sensitivity; but maybe something else is going on at the same time. Perhaps you ate more than usual or took a lot less insulin before exercising. Or perhaps you are under a lot of stress. Competitive sports can cause the body to produce adrenaline, which in turn causes the blood sugar level to rise. And some exercises, particularly those that involve short bursts of activity, just don't elicit many changes in insulin sensitivity.

Exercise may also result in a blood sugar rise if your body is dangerously low on insulin (ketones in the blood or urine usually indicate a lack of insulin). In this case, the liver will secrete extra sugar into the bloodstream, and without insulin present to help pack it into your cells, the blood sugar level rises. An insulin deficiency can occur if you forget to take a shot; if your insulin has spoiled; if your pump's infusion set comes out; or if you are coming down with an illness. Whatever the cause, do not exercise until your ketones have disappeared and your blood sugar is under better control.

Factor 4: Stress/Hormones

Last weekend I decided to stay up late and watch a scary movie. It had something to do with these super-gross vampires who get their jollies by eating the flesh of unsuspecting hotel guests. Anyway, after the final gut-wrenching, heart-pulsating scene, I decided to check my blood sugar. I'll be darned. It had risen more than 200 mg/dl (11 mmol) during the movie. With blood that sweet, I felt like the grand prize for any vampires that might happen to be in my neighborhood. Earlier, I mentioned that the liver serves as a storehouse for glucose. The liver's release of glucose depends largely on the presence of certain hormones. Of all the hormones in the body, only insulin causes the liver to take sugar out of the bloodstream and store it away. All the other hormones— including stress hormones, sex hormones, growth hormones, and most metabolic hormones—cause the liver to release glucose back into the bloodstream. Some also counteract the effects of insulin, resulting in a state of insulin resistance.

In particular, emotional stress (fear, anxiety, anger, excitement, tension) and physiological stress (illness, pain, infection, injury) cause the body to secrete a number of stress hormones into the bloodstream. These hormones are designed to prepare us for a "fight or flight" response. They make our heart rate and blood pressure increase. They make our nervous system hypersensitive. They make our eyes focus, muscles tense, temperature rise, and yes, blood sugars go up.

For those without diabetes, the stress-induced blood sugar rise is followed by an increase in insulin secretion, so the blood sugar rise is modest and momentary. For those of us with diabetes, however, stress can cause a significant and prolonged blood sugar increase.

The Little Stuff

If forgetting to put the cap back on the toothpaste or put the toilet seat down can wreck a marriage, imagine what the "little things" can do to your blood sugar!

There are countless variables that can influence blood sugar levels. Some may occur on a semiregular basis; some may occur once in a lifetime. Table 3-6 lists some of the more common "secondary influences."

⇑ Tend to Raise Blood Sugar ⇑	⇓ Tend to Lower Blood Sugar ⇓
Growth	Alcohol
Menstrual hormones	Heat/humidity
Later stages of pregnancy	Heavy brain work
Rebounds from hypoglycemia	Previous intense exercise
Gradual loss of beta cell function (type 2)	New/unusual surrounding
	Socializing
Exiting the "honeymoon" period (type 1)	Stimulating environments
	Early stages of pregnancy
Depression	Beta blockers
Weight gain	MAO inhibitors
Excessive sleeping	Nicotine patches
Caffeine	Ritalin
Steroid drugs	Stress management
Thyroid supplements	High altitude
Diuretics	
Estrogen	
Niacin	

Table 3-6: Secondary influences on blood sugar levels

See? I told you there were a lot of factors that can affect blood sugar levels. More details and methods for adjusting to these and other factors will be presented in Chapter 8.

Blood Sugar Testing Accuracy

In the movie *Wall Street,* Michael Douglas repeatedly emphasized the merits of timely, accurate information. The same holds true when managing your diabetes. Timely, accurate blood glucose readings represent the raw data used in daily management.

To ensure that your data is timely and accurate, consider the following:

1. Make sure your finger (or whatever body part you use) is clean before testing. There is no need to use alcohol, but there should not be any dirt, food, or other foreign substance on your skin. Last week, one of my patients called in a panic because her blood sugar reading was over 500 (28 mmol) for no obvious reason. Did she feel thirsty? No. Tired? No. Had to pee? No. I asked her to wash her hands and try again. The reading was 117 (6.5). It seems she was eating some chocolate just before testing and neglected to clean her hands (should have had M&Ms!).

2. Apply a sufficient drop of blood to the test strip. Some blood glucose meters will not start their countdown until enough blood is detected. Others will take a reading on whatever amount of blood is applied. If the blood sample is less than the amount required to fill the testing area, the reading may come back artificially low. It is fine to "milk" your fingertip for an adequate drop of blood, but be careful not to squeeze too hard: excessive squeezing will cause the blood sample to be mixed with interstitial fluid from below the skin, which could result in an inaccurate reading.

3. Speaking of interstitial fluid, use caution when testing body parts other than the fingertips. Blood taken from the fingertip contains just blood. "Alternate site" testing in areas such as the forearm or leg usually produces a blood

sample that is mixed with interstitial fluid. This fluid, which comes from the space between cell tissue below the skin, may not have the same glucose concentration as blood. When the blood sugar is rising (such as after meals), the glucose concentration of interstitial fluid tends to be lower than that of the blood. When the blood sugar is dropping (such as during exercise or at the peak action time of insulin), the glucose concentration of interstitial fluid tends to be higher than that of the blood. Any time you suspect that your blood sugar may be rising or dropping, it is best to test your blood sugar using only your fingertips.

4. To ensure that your test strips produce true results, be sure to properly code your meter with each new bottle or box of strips. Do not leave strips outside of their protective container for more than a few minutes, as humidity tends to affect the way they work. Do not use strips past their expiration date, and never expose your strips to extreme hot or cold temperatures.

If you are ever in doubt about the accuracy of your meter, apply a drop of control solution (included with most meters, or available from the meter manufacturer) and compare the result to the reference range. If the result is outside of the reference range, try a new package of strips. If that does not solve the problem, call the meter manufacturer and ask for a replacement meter.

4

Keys to Successful Control

"Control" Defined

Managing your diabetes should not detract from your quality of life. I define "quality diabetes management" as achieving the lowest possible **HbA1c** level without frequent or severe episodes of hypoglycemia. Occasional, mild episodes of hypoglycemia are acceptable and not dangerous for most people with diabetes. However, once low blood sugars become too frequent (more than two or three a week) or severe (causing seizures or loss of consciousness), it will be necessary to "ease back" on your targets and overall control.

For measuring your control, two types of tests are needed: The HbA1c (for measuring long-term control) and daily blood glucose readings (for assessing control at specific moments in time).

> *The Hemoglobin A1c (HbA1c) indicates the average blood glucose level over the previous 2 to 3 months.*

The HbA1c (also called a "**glycosylated hemoglobin**" or simply "A1c") provides us with an overall blood sugar average for approximately the past 2 to 3 months (see Table 4-1, below). This useful test should be completed every three months (or more often, if desired). The A1c reveals more than is shown by routine pre-meal blood sugar readings taken with your meter. As an overall average, the HbA1c indicates the degree of control before meals, after meals, and while you sleep. An A1c that comes in much higher than your pre-meal meter readings may be a sign of high after-meal or overnight blood sugars. A lower-than-expected A1c could indicate that low blood sugars are occurring without any warning. I have also found that frequent A1c testing keeps us "accountable" for our actions and serves as nice feedback for a job well done.

Given that the risk of long-term complications increases as the A1c increases, efforts should be made to keep the A1c as tight as

HbA1c	Avg. BG (mg/dl)	Avg. BG (mmol)
4	60	3.3
5	90	5.0
6	120	6.7
7	150	8.3
8	180	10.0
9	210	11.7
10	240	13.3
11	270	15.0
12	300	16.7
13	330	18.3
14	360	20.0
15	390	21.7
16	420	23.3
17	450	25.0

Table 4-1: Relationship between HbA1c and average blood glucose (BG)

To translate your HbA1c into average blood sugar, use this formula:

$$(HbA1c \times 30) - 60$$

possible. In most cases, that equates to an A1c in the 6–7% range. However, looser targets may be sought by individuals who have hypoglycemic unawareness (don't receive low blood sugar warning symptoms) or significant heart disease, as well as who work in extremely high-risk professions. Very young children who cannot communicate symptoms of hypoglycemia should also aim for a looser target. Tighter targets may be sought by women preparing for and during pregnancy, individuals planning for elective surgery, and those looking to slow or reverse existing complications.

In any case, the goal is not just the lowest average, but stability, as well. Anyone can lower his or her HbA1c level by taking too much insulin, but this would create too great a risk for frequent and severe hypoglycemia. Instead, aim to achieve a high percentage of readings within an acceptable target range.

In my experience, individuals whose pre-meal readings are within their target range less than 50% of the time should seek

	Very Tight	Typical	Looser
HbA1c Target Range	5–6%	6–7%	7–8%
Pre-Meal Target Range	60–140 (3.3–7.8)	70–160 (3.9–8.9)	80–180 (4.4–10.0)
1-Hour Post-Meal Target Range	< 160 (8.9)	< 180 (10.0)	< 200 (11.1)
Specific Pre-Meal Target	100 (5.6)	120 (6.7)	140 (7.8)

Table 4-2: Example target ranges for achieving "quality control" (mmol in parentheses)

additional self-management education or make an adjustment in their insulin dosage formulas. Between 50% and 70% "on-target" indicates fair control. More than 70% indicates very good control.

> *Successful diabetes management depends on having the right tools, skills, and attitude.*

Three Secrets to Success

Just as a chain is only as strong as its weakest link, successful diabetes management depends on three interlinked traits: tools, skills, and attitude. Having one or two just won't cut it. All three must be in place. You could have the latest cutting-edge technology at your fingertips, but without the expertise to use it properly, it would go to waste. Likewise, fancy technology and top-notch skills would fail to yield desired results without the ambition and incentive to apply them properly.

1. The Right Tools

Imagine trying to run the latest computer software on a computer built ten years ago. (Okay, so maybe you don't have to imagine!) Trying to apply the latest diabetes management techniques with yesterday's technology can be equally futile.

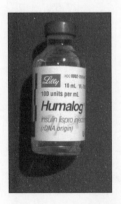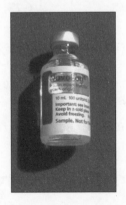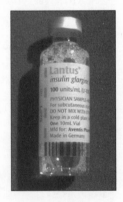

Figure 4-1: From left to right: Humalog insulin (Eli Lilly), Novolog insulin (Novo Nordisk), Lantus insulin (Aventis Pharmaceuticals)

Below are some of the "tools" that make it possible to take control of your diabetes:

The latest insulin

Today's insulin formulations are vastly superior to the insulins in use just five years ago. (Of course, by the time this goes to print, today's insulins may be equally obsolete.)

"Human" insulin (insulin that is structurally indentical to insulin produced by humans) is preferred over "animal" insulin, due to its improved absorption and tendency to elicit less of an immune response.

Insulin "analogs" are slightly altered versions of human insulin. These alterations change the timing of the insulin's action, but not its actual function.

Table 4-3 shows a summary of recommendations regarding each type of insulin.

A good insulin delivery device

If you choose to administer insulin via injections, choose a device that permits the greatest accuracy as well as convenience and flexibility.

Pens (BD, Novo Nordisk, Eli Lilly & Co.) Insulin pens are discreet, safe, fast, and simple to use, making them ideal for frequent meal/snacktime injections. Pens permit precise dosing to the nearest whole or half unit. However, the dosing accuracy depends on user technique: The pen needle must be kept in the skin for several seconds following the injection, to ensure complete insulin delivery.

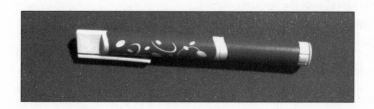

Figure 4-2: The Novo Pen Junior (Novo Nordisk) uses disposable insulin cartridges and can administer doses in half-unit increments.

Extended-Action (Basal) Insulins	Mealtime (Bolus) Insulins
☹ **NPH/Lente (Eli Lilly & Co./Novo Nordisk):** Generally not advisable for daytime usage—peak and duration of action are highly unpredictable. Tends to cause low blood sugar prior to lunch. May be useful for covering carbs eaten at lunch in the event that lunchtime injections cannot be given. May also be useful as a nighttime insulin, particularly in those who experience a marked blood sugar rise in the predawn hours.	☹ **Regular (Eli Lilly & Co./Novo Nordisk):** Not an ideal mealtime insulin. Slow onset and delayed peak often result in significant hyperglycemia after meals, followed by a prolonged blood sugar drop-off. May be useful with certain slow-digesting foods and for those with impaired digestion (gastroparesis).
☹ **Ultralente (Eli Lilly & Co. / Novo Nordisk):** Not generally advisable as either a daytime or nighttime insulin. Peak action varies considerably in terms of timing and intensity. Has a significant "upswing" and "drop-off" in action. Duration of action is highly unpredictable.	☺ **Humalog (Eli Lilly & Co.):** Excellent mealtime insulin. Rapid onset of action and early peak make it ideal for covering the blood sugar rise that occurs soon after eating carbohydrates.
☺ **Lantus (Aventis), Detemir (Novo Nordisk):** Highly recommended as basal (background) insulin. Little-to-no peak activity. Duration of action is fairly consistent.	☺ **Novolog (Novo Nordisk):** Same benefits as lispro. Aspart's "buffered" solution makes it preferred for use in insulin pumps.

Table 4-3: Recommendations regarding insulin use

Pens come either prefilled or with disposable insulin cartridges. The disposable needles used on insulin pens are thinner and sharper than traditional syringe needles, and hence are more comfortable. Select a pen needle length that is appropriate for your body type. If you are very lean, choose a short pen needle (5–8 mm). If you have adequate body fat, choose a longer needle (10–12 mm).

Syringes (BD) When choosing insulin syringes, select the smallest size possible given your usual dose. This allows for the greatest dosage accuracy. 100–unit syringes (which have markings every 2 units) would not be appropriate for someone on a relatively low dose who wants to be able to give insulin in whole or half units. Even 50-unit syringes (which have single-unit markings) are less than ideal for someone who wants to do half-unit dosing. Syringes are now available with half-unit markings. Use these unless you require more than 25 units per injection.

As far as the needle itself, thinner is almost always better. Thin needles (needles with a high gauge—30 or more) are usually more comfortable and lead to less scarring than thicker needles. The optimal needle *length* depends on your body type. If you are overweight, "short" (5–8 mm) needles may not inject the insulin deep enough to achieve proper absorption. If you are lean, standard-length needles (10–12 mm) may accidentally inject the insulin into muscle. This can cause pain, bruising, and accelerated insulin absorption.

If you have plenty of body fat, use standard-length needles. If you have difficulty pinching up an inch or more of body fat, use short needles.

Air Injectors (Activa, Antares) Air injection is another mechanism for infusing insulin below the skin. Air injectors use pressurized air to create an insulin "mist" that travels through the pores of the skin at a high speed. When used properly, these devices can be almost painless and may help those with severe needle phobias. Used improperly, they can cause bruising, scarring, and inaccurate insulin dosing.

Air injectors are designed to be used only with fast-acting mealtime insulin. Because of the dispersion of insulin below the skin, the insulin may begin working sooner and peak earlier than insulin given by syringe or pen.

Pumps (Animas, Dana, Deltec, Disetronic, MiniMed, Nipro)
Insulin pumps were first developed in the 1970s, as scientists and physicians looked for a way to copy the world's best blood sugar control device: a healthy pancreas.

The insulin pump copies the human pancreas by releasing small amounts of fast-acting insulin (in tenths or hundreths of a unit) every few minutes. This is called **basal** insulin. When food is eaten, the user programs the pump to deliver a larger quantity of insulin fairly quickly. This is called **bolus** insulin.

Insulin pumps are the size of beepers and contain a cartridge filled with fast-acting insulin. They have a sensitive motor that turns very gradually, to push insulin from the cartridge through a tube and into your body.

It is important to note that the pump does not control blood

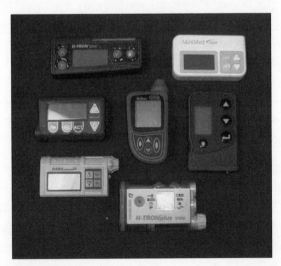

Figure 4-3: Insulin pumps

sugars automatically. It takes a skilled, educated, and motivated user to use the pump properly and benefit to the fullest.

Selecting a pump is a matter of personal preference. All pumps have a set of basic features that allow safe, precise delivery of basal and bolus insulin. Beyond that, a slew of bells and whistles, ranging from vibrate options to built-in dosage calculators, can be found. Shop around for the pump with the features you desire. A list of manufacturers and Web sites, and comparisons of the various pumps can be found in Chapter 10.

A modern meter (Abbott, Bayer, Lifescan, Roche, Therasense)

Because diabetes management requires frequent blood sugar testing, look for a meter that is fast (some take as little as 5 seconds), simple to use (fewer "steps" means less chance for user error), downloadable (and with substantial memory), and requiring very little blood (1 microliter or less is ideal).

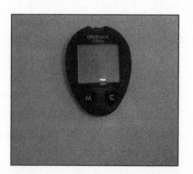 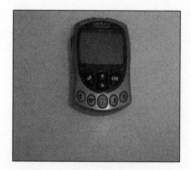

Figure 4-4: The Ultra (left) and UltraSmart (right) meters from Lifescan use very small blood samples and are very fast.

With the advent of "alternate-site" meters (meters that can perform a test on blood samples from places other than the sensitive fingertips), virtually pain-free blood glucose testing has become a reality. However, be aware that alternate-site testing rarely works with meters that require 1 microliter of blood or more. Also, readings taken from the arm or leg may lag several minutes behind readings taken from the fingertips. This is because blood samples taken from the arm or leg are usually mixed with *interstitial fluid*—the fluid that surrounds cells and tissues below the skin. It usually takes 10 to 15 minutes for changes in blood sugar to be reflected in the interstitial fluid, so samples taken from the arm or leg may not match the blood sugar exactly. If you suspect that your blood sugar is dropping quickly (after exercise, or if you feel hypoglycemic) or rising quickly (after meals), blood taken from the fingertip will provide a more accurate reading than blood taken from alternate sites.

Be sure that the meter you use provides *plasma* glucose readings, rather than whole blood readings. Lab equipment is calibrated to measure plasma glucose, which is essentially blood without the blood cells. Whole blood glucose levels are generally 10–15% lower than plasma glucose levels. Most modern meters provide plasma-calibrated readings. Meters made prior to the 1990s may be providing whole blood measurements. If in doubt, call the number on the back of your meter and ask the manufacturer.

It would also be beneficial to have more than one meter. Some meter companies will send you an extra meter at no charge, assuming that you will continue to purchase and use their test strips. Personally, I keep a meter in each of the places where I do the most testing: bedside, kitchen, desk at work, and gym bag. I don't keep one in the car because test strips can spoil easily at very high and low temperatures. Instead, I keep one in my briefcase for testing before I drive home.

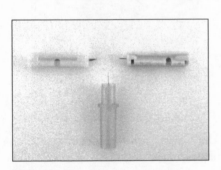

Figure 4-5: Using an adjustable lancet pen and thin lancets (such as the Ultra-Fine 33 Gauge Lancet from BD, pictured at the bottom) makes blood glucose testing infinitely more comfortable.

A supportive health care team

We've all heard the saying, "A lawyer who defends himself has an idiot for a client." The same goes for anyone who neglects to call on the expertise of health care professionals for proper diabetes care.

Surrounding yourself with a quality health care team is like putting together a winning basketball team. You need scorers who can create good shots; defenders who can shut down opposing players; ballhandlers who can find the open man; and role players who can hustle, rebound, and do the "little things" to help the team win.

One approach is to go with a "preassembled" team of diabetes professionals. The American Diabetes Association keeps a list of "recognized diabetes self-management programs" that feature a variety of diabetes care specialists. Although there are many quality providers not included on the list, the programs on the list have all been recognized by the American Diabetes Association for meeting national standards for diabetes education. For an updated list, go to www.diabetes.org/education/edustate2.asp, or call 800–342–2383.

Once your team is in place, is your job done? Hardly. Many teams have failed to win championships because they have a bunch of high-priced stars who refuse to be "team players." As a coach, you must put together the best combination of players and play to their strengths.

Your health care lineup should include:

The Physican—Your physician is the center on your health care team. He or she is ultimately responsible for diagnosing and treating your diabetes, screening for complications, prescribing the necessary tests and medications, and making sure that your control is on target. As a center, the physician oversees the activities of the other players and is ultimately accountable for making sure you receive the right treatment.

Of course, different physicians have different levels of expertise in treating diabetes. **Endocrinologists** typically have the most experience and skill in diabetes care. However, some endocrinologists specialize in treating type 2/non-insulin-using diabetes, whereas others focus on people who use insulin.

Internal medicine doctors (internists) usually treat a variety of chronic health conditions, diabetes being just one of them. Some internists have a great deal of expertise in treating diabetes; others tend to refer their diabetic patients elsewhere. General practitioners (family doctors) typically treat many short-term and long-term illnesses and have only a basic understanding of how to manage diabetes. However, any physician can provide excellent diabetes care if he or she calls on the resources of other health professionals to help patients with their control.

Now, here's a practical question: What would you do as coach of a basketball team if a player were not performing up to standards? Chances are, you would try to coach him or her through it, by talking it over and offering some suggestions. If that didn't work, or if the player refused to be coached, you would probably cut the player or make a trade.

It is your right—and responsibility—to switch doctors if you are not satisfied with the service you are receiving.

You might want to consider switching to another physician if your doctor:

- does not explain things in a way you can understand;

- won't answer your questions or refer you to someone who can;

- fails to perform the necessary screenings for diabetic complications;

- does not order the proper lab tests or provide your prescriptions in a timely manner;

- will not recognize the importance of your cultural traditions when devising your diabetes management plan;

- refuses to refer you to a specialist such as an endocrinolo-gist, podiatrist, or dietitian;

- for unclear or unsubstantiated reasons, denies you access to current technology such as an insulin pump or moni-toring device; and/or

- does not recognize the importance of obtaining tight blood sugar control, or has not been successful at helping you improve your control.

The Certified Diabetes Educator—The point guard on your team is the Certified Diabetes Educator (CDE). A CDE is often a nurse but can also be a dietitian, pharmacist, exercise physiologist, physician, mental health counselor, or anyone in the health care field with advanced training in diabetes management.

A CDE (Certified Diabetes Educator) can teach you all you need to know about diabetes self-management, as well as guide you through the issues of day-to-day living with diabetes.

In many cases, a CDE will be able to teach and guide you through the issues of living day-to-day with diabetes. Whereas a physician often has limited time to spend with you and may not be a particularly good teacher, a CDE will take the time to teach you the right ways to self-manage your diabetes.

To locate a CDE in your area, talk to your doctor or con-tact the American Association of Diabetes Educators at 800–338–3633 (www.aadenet.org) and ask for the CDE referral program.

The Dietitian—Any time you check your blood sugar, what and when you ate will almost always have a major influence. Working with a professional dietary counselor can make the difference between good control and no control at all. A registered dietitian (RD, preferably also a CDE) will work with you to increase your knowledge and skills in carbohydrate counting, weight control, sports nutrition, special occasion dining, alcohol safety, and dietary management of conditions such as hypertension, celiac disease, and elevated cholesterol.

To find a registered dietitian specializing in diabetes, contact the American Dietetic Association at 800–877–1600 or www.eatright.org/public (click on the "find a nutrition professional" icon).

The Counselor—With all the pressure placed on people with diabetes to manage blood sugar levels while taking care of everything else in their lives, a mental health counselor can be a valuable member of your health care team. Mental health professionals (social workers, psychologists, and psychiatrists) can help with issues such as depression, eating disorders, sleep disturbances, obsessive/compulsive behaviors, anxieties, relationship difficulties, financial hardship, and job discrimination.

In most cases, psychological issues must be dealt with before you can expect to do an effective job at controlling your diabetes. So, if you are experiencing problems that are interfering with your ability to take good care of yourself, a mental health counselor might be the first and best person to contact. To find a counselor, contact your health insurance plan for a list of participating providers in your area.

The Exercise Specialist—Exercise is a hot topic in diabetes because of all the benefits it has to offer. However, you can also get yourself in hot water if you exercise improperly. Severe hypoglycemia, acute injuries, and worsening of diabetic complications are among the risks faced by people with diabetes who exercise.

An exercise physiologist is a health professional who understands the physical, psychological, and metabolic effects of exercise. He or she can help you design an exercise plan, adjust insulin doses to prevent hypoglycemia, manage blood sugars during sports/competitive activity, and reduce your risk for injuries and other complications.

Look for an exercise physiologist with at least a master's degree. An exercise physiologist who is also a CDE may be your best option.

The Role Players—Given the complexity of diabetes and the many organ systems that are affected, it would be wise to include a few other specialists on your health team. These include a podiatrist for preventive foot care and treatment of foot problems, an ophthalmologist for routine eye exams and treatment of eye disorders, and a dentist for ongoing tooth/gum care.

2. The Right Skills

Modern technology is useless without the know-how to utilize it properly. I've seen people with the latest, cutting-edge diabetes paraphernalia who were completely clueless as to how to manage their blood sugar levels. High-tech devices are nice, but ultimately, it is your skill in diabetes management that gets you the control you want.

The following are skills that everyone using insulin should adopt:

Frequent Blood Sugar Testing

From my experience, patients who test their blood sugar levels four to eight times daily tend to have the best overall control. Less frequent testing leaves you open to running at high blood sugar levels for long stretches of time, and much more frequent testing often results in overcompensation for high readings and frequent hypoglycemic reactions.

The best times to check blood sugars are:

- before each meal and snack (being careful not to eat too frequently);

- prior to exercise;

- prior to driving or performing potentially hazardous work;

- before going to bed;

- (occasionally) an hour after meals (to assess post-meal control); and

- (occasionally) in the middle of the night, to ensure that your long-acting/basal insulin is holding you steady while you sleep.

From a procedural standpoint, to help ensure the accuracy of your readings, be sure to use test strips prior to their expiration date; keep the strips sealed in their bottle or foil wrapping; and be sure to apply enough blood to cover the test area completely.

Because you will be checking your blood sugar frequently, here are a few hints for making your blood sugar testing more comfortable:

- Use the thinnest-gauge lancet you can find. Presently, 33-gauge lancets (BD) are the thinnest on the market (the higher the gauge, the thinner the lancet). Thin lancets are less painful and cause less scarring than thicker lancets.

- Use an adjustable-depth lancing pen (BD, Palco Labs) and set it at the lightest possible setting that still produces a sufficient blood sample.

- Use the sides of your fingertips rather than the tips themselves.

- Alternate-site testing is almost always less painful than fingertip testing, as long as the readings are taken at times when blood sugar levels are holding fairly steady.

Carbohydrate Gram Counting

As mentioned in the previous chapter, carbohydrates are the primary blood sugar–raising elements in the diet. All carbohydrates (simple and complex), with the exception of fiber, convert into blood glucose fairly rapidly. Thus, having the ability to quantify the carbohydrates in our meals and snacks is of the utmost importance.

For starters, carbohydrates should always be counted in grams. This is the most precise and practical way to count carbs. Using carb "choices" or "exchanges" tends to make things more complex but less precise.

To make the transition from "exchanges" to grams, use Table 4-4, below. Simply add the amount of carbohydrates you are getting from each exchange, and you have your carb total for your meal.

In other words, a meal containing 2 breads, 2 fruits, a milk and 3 meats contains $(2 \times 15) + (2 \times 15) + (1 \times 12) + (3 \times 0)$, or 72 grams of carbohydrate. Just make sure you have the right portion sizes for each exchange. For example, one ordinary banana may be 1, 1½, or 2 fruit exchanges, depending on the size.

1 "Bread" Exchange	=	15 grams carb
1 "Fruit" Exchange	=	15 grams carb
1 "Milk" Exchange	=	12 grams carb
1 "Vegetable" Exchange	=	5 grams carb
1 "Meat" Exchange	=	0 grams carb
1 "Fat" Exchange	=	0 grams carb

Table 4-4: Converting exchanges to grams carb

Count all the carbs equally. True, there are some subtle differences in terms of how quickly different carbohydrates raise the blood sugar, but all carbs (except for fiber) eventually turn into blood glucose, so count them all the same. For example, 12 grams of carbohydrate from milk will raise the blood sugar more slowly than 12 grams of carbohydrate from bread, but after a few hours, the total rise will be equal.

If you consume a food high in fiber, such as whole grain bread, beans, or bran cereal, you may not see as much of a blood sugar rise as you might expect. Fiber is a carbohydrate that does not digest and hence does not raise the blood sugar. When consuming foods that contain more than 3 grams of fiber, subtract the fiber grams from the total carbohydrate. For example, a high-fiber cereal that contains 11 grams of fiber and 31 grams of total carbohydrate would be counted as 20 grams of carb (31 minus 11).

> *Fiber is a carbohydrate that does not digest and hence does not raise the blood sugar.*

There are a number of techniques for counting carbs. The first and most basic is label reading.

All food labels are required to list the serving size, total carbohydrate content, and carbohydrate breakdown (note that food labels include the fiber in the total carbohydrate even though fiber does not convert into blood sugar):

Sugars (simple carbohydrate)
+ Starch/other (complex carbohydrate)
+ Fiber
_____
Total carbohydrate

Figure 4-6 shows a sample food label: A serving of Gloopers (½ cup) contains 20 grams of total carbohydrate. If you consume a full cup, you would have 40 grams of carb.

"**Sugar alcohols**" such as sorbitol, mannitol, and xylitol are also included in the total carbohydrates. Sugar alcohols are used as sweeteners in many "sugar-free" foods. Although slow to act, sugar alcohols will raise blood sugar as much as other carbohydrates.

Another tool for carbohydrate gram counting is a nutrient guide: There are many pamphlets, books, and Web sites that list the carbohydrate content of various foods. Some cover specific categories such as restaurant food or ethnic food; others cover a wide range of commonly consumed foods.

Some of my favorites are available at my Web site: (www.integrateddiabetes.com). They include the following:

• *The Doctor's Pocket Calorie, Fat & Carbohydrate Counter* by

Delicious, Chocolatey Gloopers

Serving Size ½ cup (1 oz)
Servings per Container 8

Nutrition Facts
Amount per Serving

Calories 150	
Total Fat 6g	10%
Saturated Fat 5g	25%
Sodium 120 mg	5%
Total Carbohydrate 20g	7%
Sugar 12g	
Protein 2g	3%

Figure 4-6: Delicious, Chocolatey Gloopers

Family Health Publications: Compact paperback with a very comprehensive listing of carb content of common foods, ethnic foods, restaurant foods, and beverages. Indexed for easy searching. Also available in electronic form for electronic organizers. $6.99 (call 949–642–8500, or go to www.CalorieKing.com)

- *Nutrition in the Fast Lane* by Franklin Publishing: Slim brochure containing nutritional content for most menu items from 39 popular restaurant chains. $4.95 + s/h (call 800–634–1993)

- *Fast Food Facts* by Marion Franz of the International Diabetes Center: Complete nutrient listings for dozens of convenience restaurants. $9.95 (call 888–637–2675 or go to www.idcpublishing.com)

- *Counting Calories & Carbs* by Novo Nordisk Pharmaceuticals: Brochure listing approximate calorie and carb content for many common foods. Free (call 800–382–7265, enter "0" to reach an attendant)

- *Nutrition Facts Desk Reference* by Dr. Art Ulene: Large, comprehensive guide to food nutrients. $18 (available at most major bookstores)

- *Food Values* by Jean Pennington: A comprehensive guide to food nutrients. $30 (available at most major bookstores)

A somewhat more sophisticated technique for counting carbs is portion estimation. This method is particularly useful when dining out or enjoying foods that vary in size, such as whole fruits or baked goods.

Portion estimation involves using a common object such as your fist or a deck of cards to determine the approximate size of a particular food item. Then, the carb count is determined based on the typical carb content for a standard size of that item.

Common "measuring devices":

Soda can = 1½ cups
Adult's fist = approx. 1 cup
Large handful = approx. 1 cup
Tennis ball = approx. ½ cup
Cupped hand = approx. ½ cup
Child's fist = approx. ½ cup
Adult's spread hand = approx. 8" diameter
Adult's palm = approx. 4" diameter

Approximate carb counts for standard portion sizes:

Potato ≈ 30g/cup
Pasta (w/sauce) ≈ 35g/cup
Rice (boiled) ≈ 50g/cup

Sticky rice ≈ 75g/cup
Salad/raw vegetables ≈ 5g/cup
Cooked vegetables ≈ 10g/cup
Rolls ≈ 25g/cup
Dense bread (bagel/soft pretzel) ≈ 50g/cup
Fruit ≈ 20g/cup
Ice cream ≈ 35g/cup
Cake/muffin/pie ≈ 45g/cup
Pretzels ≈ 25g/cup
Chips ≈ 15g/cup
Popcorn ≈ 5g/cup
Cereal ≈ 25g/cup
Milk ≈ 12g/cup
Juice, soda ≈ 30g/cup
Sport drink ≈ 15g/cup
Sub sandwich rolls ≈ 8g/inch
Pizza ≈ 40g/8" diameter (round)
Pizza ≈ 30g/closed hand (slice)
Cookie ≈ 20g/4" diameter
Pancake ≈ 15g/4" diameter
Tortilla ≈ 15g/8" diameter

For example, an adult's fist is equal to about a 1-cup portion. If a cup of boiled rice contains 50 grams of carbohydrates and you consume 1½ fist-size portions of pasta, you will have eaten about 75 grams of carbohydrates. Three large handfuls of chips will contain 3 × 15, or 45 grams of carbohydrates. A 10" submarine sandwich will contain 10 × 8, or 80 g carb.

The most precise technique for counting carbs involves using carb factors. By weighing the portion of food that you plan to eat on a gram scale and multiplying the weight by the food's carb factor, you will obtain a precise carb count.

A carb factor is actually the percentage of a food's weight that is carbohydrate. For example, apples have a carb factor of 0.13, which means that 13% of an apple's weight is carbohydrate. If an apple weighs 120 grams, the carb content is 120 × 0.13, or 15.6 grams.

> A *carb factor* represents the percentage of a food's weight that is *carbohydrate*.

For an abbreviated list of carb factors, see Appendix A.

For a detailed list of carb factors for more than 6,000 foods, go to www.friendswithdiabetes.org/carb_factor.html.

To figure out the carb factor for any packaged food item, simply divide the total carbohydrate for a single serving (in grams) by the weight of a single serving. For example, if a serving of pastry contains 60 grams of carb and weighs 150 grams, its carb factor is 60/150, or 0.40.

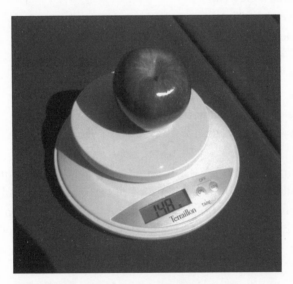

Figure 4-7: Using an electronic food scale along with carbohydrate factors allows us to determine the exact carb content of almost any food.

Insulin Dosage Adjustment

Self-adjustment of insulin doses is a primary component of "Thinking Like a Pancreas." Short-term insulin doses should be adjusted based on:

- Pre-meal/pre-snack blood sugar levels

- Carbohydrate intake

- Physical activity

- Moods/stress/hormone levels

- Illness and medications

In addition, adjustments should be made to your overall insulin plan in the event of recurrent hypoglycemia or hyperglycemia that occurs repeatedly at similar times of day.

Insulin dosage adjustment and overall plan changes will be the focal point of the next three chapters of this book.

Record-Keeping and Analysis

By keeping organized, detailed records and analyzing them on a regular basis, you can gain much better control of your diabetes.

Any good record-keeping system begins with blood glucose readings. If you take two or more injections of insulin daily or use an insulin pump, you should be testing your blood sugar at least four times daily—upon waking, before the midday meal, before dinner, and before bedtime/evening snack. Even if you don't take insulin at each of these times, the blood sugar information is needed to determine when you might be rising or falling. For example, if the blood sugar is high at dinner, the lunch reading allows us to determine whether the rise took place in the morning or the afternoon.

For those taking insulin once daily, blood sugar readings should be taken twice daily—at least while control is being fine-tuned. Ideally, the readings should be taken at two meals in a row and "rotated" from day to day. For example, on day one, test before breakfast and lunch. On day two, test before lunch and dinner. On day three, test at dinner and bedtime. Then repeat the process from day one. This approach lets you see when blood sugar levels may be rising or falling.

Blood sugar readings by themselves are not of much use, unless they are all running high or low. For most of us, that just isn't the case. It is necessary to figure out *why* the readings went high or low. Was it caused by too much or too little food? Improper insulin/medication types or doses? Changes in physical activity? Stress or illness?

> *A good set of written records should include blood sugar readings, as well as the main factors that affect blood sugars—insulin doses, grams of carb, physical activity, and stressful events.*

To figure out why your blood sugar levels vary, record the amount of insulin taken; the grams of carbohydrate consumed at each meal and snack; the type and length of exercise and other physical activities performed (such as housework, yardwork, shopping, and extended walking); as well as stresses that tend to affect blood sugars (such as illnesses, menstrual cycles, emotional events, and hypoglycemic episodes).

For those checking blood sugars twice a day, try to record the pertinent information (insulin, carbs, activity, stress) between the two tests. For example, if testing prior to breakfast and lunch, record all carbs/activities/insulin from the time you wake up until just before lunch.

To get the most from your record-keeping, organize the information so that it will be easy to analyze. Charts like those in Appendix C have been very helpful to my patients. These forms are also available in a printable form at my Web site: www.integrated-diabetes.com.

I find it helpful to have the times of day lined up in columns so that I can go through them and quickly assess how many readings are above, below, and within my target range. This gives me and my patients the ability to interpret the data effectively.

Learning how to interpret your self-monitoring records is also essential. Otherwise, your records are nothing more than pieces of paper with a bunch of numbers and little blood spots on them.

Are you consistently high or low at certain times of day? Does physical activity have an immediate or delayed effect? Do certain types of foods always seem to make your blood sugars rise? Is stress impacting your control? Every time you make a sensible adjustment based on your records, your control will get a little bit better.

Review your own records on a weekly or bimonthly basis. Keep track of how many readings are above, below, and within your target range for each time of day that you test. If more than 25% of your readings are coming in above target at a certain time of day, or more than 10% are coming in low, changes to your insulin program or dosing formulas are probably in order. Because low blood sugars can sometimes result in high readings a few hours later, it is usually best to deal with the low blood sugar problems before addressing the high.

> *Frequent high or low readings at a certain time of day indicate a need for a change in your insulin program. It is advisable to address the low blood sugar problem before trying to adjust for the highs.*

Before meeting with your physician or diabetes educator, prepare a summary of your control. This can be done manually (by tallying your readings by hand) or by downloading your blood glucose meter to a computer and printing out a modal day and summary statistics. Virtually all meter manufacturers have software and cables available for their customers. Call the customer service number on the back of your meter to order. Once again, if you are frequently high or low at a specific time of day, look for possible causes and propose a solution at your appointment. It never hurts to get a professional

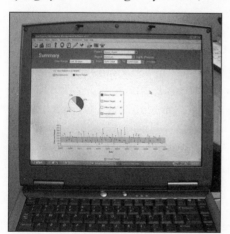

Figure 4-8: Downloading your meter to a computer can reveal important patterns and trends.

opinion! Be sure to bring all of your blood glucose meters to your appointment, and make certain that the time and date are set correctly on each.

3. The Right Attitude (You can lead a diabetic to insulin, but you can't make him inject)

A week doesn't go by that I don't come across someone (young or old) who has everything he or she needs to manage his or her diabetes—the latest high-tech toys; a great plan; all the self-management education, training, and support in the world. Everything . . . except the right attitude.

> *Keeping your diabetes in control is what* enables *you to enjoy life and* fulfill all your other obligations.

A healthy approach to living with diabetes is just as important as the tools and skills outlined above. Perhaps even more important. See how you fare in the following areas:

Determination

Exactly where does managing diabetes rank in your set of personal priorities? Although nobody would expect you to place your diabetes care above the immediate well-being of your family, it should hold a prominent place in your life. And with good reason. Managing your diabetes *enables* you to fulfill all your other obligations and enjoy all that life has to offer. Think about it: If your diabetes is not in control, how will it affect you at work? At school? At home? In bed? At the gym?

Your diabetes control affects virtually every aspect of your life. With poor control, you may be able to *function*—but not *perform*. With prolonged poor control, your health can deteriorate to the point that functioning becomes impossible.

Don't let anything get in the way of managing your diabetes properly. That includes costs. If your insurance company is unwilling to pay for a product or service that you feel you need to manage your diabetes, fight the company on it. Contact your state attorney general's office if your insurance company is not complying with state regulations regarding coverage for diabetes supplies and education. And if necessary, pay out of pocket. You simply cannot put a price on your health.

Persistence

Michael Jordan was perhaps the greatest basketball player of all time. A prolific scorer, tenacious defender, and fierce competitor, MJ managed to win six NBA championships despite being "undersized" (he was a mere 6'6") and lacking a dominant supporting cast. But did you know that Michael "Air" Jordan, icon of the basketball world, was cut from his high school basketball team as a freshman? Had Michael chosen to throw in the towel and concentrate on baseball or (heaven forbid) his studies, he would have deprived himself and the rest of the world of his amazing natural talents.

Persistence is a valuable trait in many aspects of life. From work to dating to basketball, persistence usually pays off in a big way. This is certainly evident when it comes to managing diabetes. Given the relentless nature of this disease, it takes tremendous persistence to manage over the long term. Over the course of your life with diabetes, there will be countless setbacks. When they occur, *do not give up*. If possible, use those setbacks as an opportunity to re-focus and fine-tune your management strategies.

Of course, it is reasonable to take a mini-vacation from time to time—so long as you maintain a level of care that keeps you out of harm's way and you get back on track reasonably soon. I have many patients who take a few days each month to ease back on their usual diet, exercise, and record-keeping routine. They still take their insulin and check their blood sugar, but the short break serves as a nice refresher.

Discipline

Despite being a general pain in the neck, some good things come from having diabetes. We can get seated in restaurants faster. We know how to take better care of our bodies. And we also can develop a healthy sense of discipline.

Being disciplined does not mean living like an emotionless robot. It means maintaining a desired course of action even in the face of distraction and adversity. Maybe not all the time, but certainly most of the time.

People who are disciplined about their diet, avoiding unnecessary and frequent snacks, tend to achieve much better blood sugar control.

For example, I have found that people who are disciplined about their diet tend to maintain much better control of their diabetes than people who eat inconsistently and erratically. Frequent snacking, in particular, can wreck a person's diabetes control and lead to unwanted weight gain. For that reason, it is best to space meals and snacks at least 3 to 4 hours apart. Here's why:

Imagine that you are on a boat that has sprung a leak. Rather than plugging the leak, you start bailing out the water. No matter how fast you bail, water keeps rushing in, and the water level in the boat never goes down.

The same thing happens to blood sugar levels when you eat too frequently. Blood sugars always rise temporarily after eating, coming back down to normal approximately 3 hours later (assuming that fast-acting insulin is given with the food). If you eat every hour or 2, the blood sugar level is constantly at a high "after eating" level. Just when it starts coming down toward normal, more food hits your bloodstream and causes the level to rise once again. However, if you eat and then wait at least 3 hours before eating again, the blood sugar has a chance to return to normal. It's like plugging the hole in the boat before you start bailing.

Another benefit of waiting at least 3 hours between meals and snacks is that you can be reasonably sure that the fast-acting insulin you gave previously is just about finished working. Otherwise, you may start overlapping your insulin doses and wind up with a serious low blood sugar a few hours later.

Another area where discipline is valuable is exercise. Physical activity can amplify the effects of insulin for up to 48 hours. Those who maintain a consistent pattern of exercise usually have predictable insulin action. Those who are "off and on" in regard to exercise usually have a hard time predicting how hard their insulin will work.

For example, if you're the "weekend warrior" type—lots of activity on the weekends, very little during the week—you will probably find that your insulin sensitivity varies considerably. You may be more prone to unexpected lows on Saturday, Sunday, and Monday, as your sensitivity to insulin is very high. Then, you might see unusual highs on Tuesday, Wednesday, Thursday, and Friday, as you lose insulin sensitivity and your insulin fails to achieve the desired effects. By comparison, someone who exercises consistently throughout the week will have a fairly stable level of insulin sensitivity and hence more consistent insulin action.

People who are disciplined about keeping written records, checking blood sugar levels, counting carbohydrates, calculating insulin doses accurately (and *remembering* to take their insulin), and seeing health care providers regularly also tend to show better quality blood sugar control over the long term.

Acceptance

Despite your best efforts, you will not be in perfect control of your diabetes all the time. That's okay. If a baseball player went to pieces every time he failed to get a hit, we would have a lot of .300 hitters sitting in the dugout crying.

Set your expectations at a realistic level. Using the "acceptable range" chart at the beginning of the chapter might serve as a good starting point. And remember, even the best-controlled patients are still "out of range" 20 to 30% of the time.

Also, accept your own personal limitations. Trying to change too much all at once usually leads to burnout. Make a list of all the things you could be doing to improve your control, and prioritize them. Then try to implement one at a time.

For example, if you are just getting started in the pursuit of intensive diabetes management, you might try implementing one change each week, as follows:

Week 1: Start checking your blood sugar level before each meal and snack, and writing down the results.

Week 2: Learn to adjust your insulin doses appropriately based on your pre-meal/pre-snack blood sugar levels.

Week 3: Begin looking up the carb counts in your foods and writing them down, along with your blood sugars and insulin doses.

Week 4: Learn to adjust your insulin doses based on carbohydrate intake.

Week 5: Start getting some daily exercise, and add that to your written records.

Week 6: Learn to adjust your insulin doses based on physical activity.

Keep in mind that your diabetes records—including blood sugar levels—are simply *information* that can be used by you and your health care team for making competent decisions and fine-tuning your management plan. They are not meant to pass judgment on you as a person. As I tell many of my patients, "Any information is good information—regardless of the numbers."

Finally, memorize the Serenity Prayer. Don't misunderstand: I am not a very religious person. But I know when something makes sense. The Serenity Prayer reminds us that not everything is within our control. To fret over things beyond your control is a waste of time and effort. Instead, concentrate on the things you do have some control over. We may not have the final say over what each blood sugar reading is, but we can improve our odds of a decent reading if we do the right things.

A little bit of luck (or help from above) wouldn't hurt, either.

THE SERENITY PRAYER
God, grant me the serenity to accept the things I cannot change,
the courage to change the things I can,
and the wisdom to know the difference.

Keys to Control Checklist

The right tools:
___ The latest insulin
___ A good insulin delivery device
___ A modern blood glucose meter
___ A supportive health-care team

The right skills:
___ Frequent blood insulin testing
___ Carbohydrate gram counting
___ Insulin dosage adjustment
___ Record-keeping and analysis

The right attitude:
___ Determination
___ Persistence
___ Discipline
___ Acceptance

5

The Basal/Bolus Approach

So, YOU'VE GOT ALL your key components in place. Your home is littered with used test strips. Your carb counting skills rival those of the diabetes gods. You're even keeping written records for the first time in your life. Now all you need is the right insulin plan to make it pay off.

If you're going to think like a pancreas, your insulin program should include the two Bs: "basal" or "background" insulin, along with "boluses" or "bunches" of insulin at mealtimes.

Basal Insulin

Every few minutes, a healthy pancreas secretes a small amount of insulin into the bloodstream. This **basal insulin** is necessary to provide the body's cells with a continuous supply of sugar to burn for energy. Because the liver is secreting sugar into the bloodstream continuously, a complete lack of insulin would result in a sharp rise in blood sugar levels.

The level of basal insulin should match the liver's secretion of sugar throughout the day and night. In the absence of food and exercise, the basal insulin level should hold the blood sugar fairly steady.

> *The basal insulin level should be matched to the liver's normal secretion of sugar. Basal insulin is needed to hold the blood sugar level steady between meals and during sleep.*

Each person's basal insulin requirement is unique. Typically, basal insulin needs are highest during the night and early morning, and lowest in the middle of the day. This is due to the production of blood sugar–raising hormones during the night, and enhanced sensitivity to insulin that comes with daytime physical activity. Table 5-1, below, shows typical basal insulin requirements for people with insulin-dependent diabetes. The chart is based on data from several hundred insulin pump users whose basal insulin levels were carefully adjusted and fine-tuned:

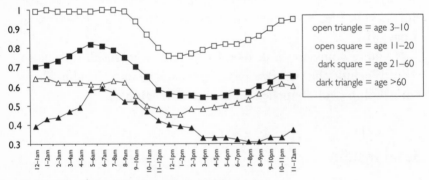

open triangle = age 3–10
open square = age 11–20
dark square = age 21–60
dark triangle = age >60

Table 5-1: Typical basal insulin requirements

Although no significant differences are found in the basal insulin requirements for men versus women, age does play a significant role. During a person's growth years (prior to age 21), basal insulin needs tend to be relatively high throughout the night, drop through the morning hours, and gradually increase from noon to midnight. Most adults (age 21+) exhibit an abrupt increase in basal insulin needs during the early morning hours, followed by a drop-off until noontime, a low/flat level in the afternoon, and a gradual increase in the evening. This peak in basal insulin requirements during the early morning hours is commonly referred to as a "**dawn phenomenon.**"

> Dawn phenomenon refers to an increase in basal insulin needs in the early morning hours. It is caused by the increased production of certain hormones (growth hormone, cortisol) during this time.

The magnitude and pattern of basal insulin requirements reflect the amount and timing of cortisol and growth hormone secretion within each age category. The youngest group (age ≤10) requires approximately 40% less basal insulin than those 11–20, but the 24-hour pattern of peaks and valleys is remarkably similar. Likewise, the oldest group (age>60) requires approximately 33% less basal insulin that those in the 21–60 age group, but with a similar 24-hour pattern.

Basal insulin can be supplied in a variety of ways. Intermediate-acting insulins (NPH and Lente) taken once daily will usually provide background insulin around the clock, albeit at much higher levels 4 to 8 hours after injection and at much lower levels at 16 to 24 hours. Long-acting insulin (Ultralente) provides basal insulin for 24 to 36 hours, but usually with a "peak" at 8 to 16 hours, followed by an extended drop-off in action. Basal insulins (Lantus and Detemir) offer relatively peakless insulin levels for approximately 24 hours. Insulin pumps deliver rapid-acting insulin in small pulses throughout the day and night. With a pump, the basal insulin level can be adjusted and fine-tuned to match the body's ebb and flow in basal insulin needs.

The following four tables illustrate the action of basal insulin using various types of insulin programs:

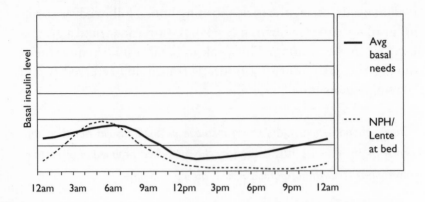

Table 5-2: Basal Option 1: NPH or Lente once daily, at bedtime

The advantage of this program is the peak that occurs during the pre-dawn hours. The disadvantages include the unpredictability of the peak, and the potential for daytime/evening blood sugar rises as the tail of insulin action fails to meet the liver's production of glucose.

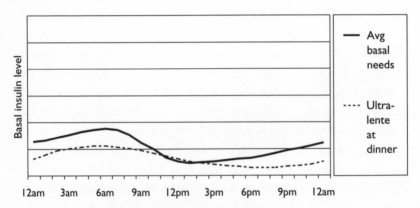

Table 5-3: Basal Option 2: Ultralente once daily, at dinner

The advantage of the Ultralente program is the gradual peak during the night along with a fairly steady flow of basal insulin throughout the 24-hour time period. The disadvantages include absorption inconsistencies, potential blood sugar rises during the night (due to the lack of a substantial peak), and potential for blood sugar rises during the evening, as the insulin wears off. In many instances, Ultralente can last

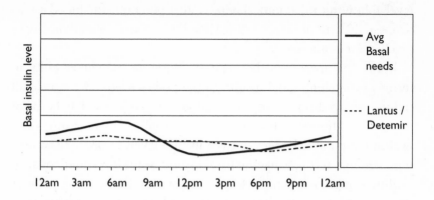

Table 5-4: Basal Option 3: Lantus once only at dinnertime or Detemir twice daily (at breakfast and dinnertime)

up to 36 hours—resulting in an overlap when the injections are taken 24 hours apart. This, too, can cause erratic and unpredictable insulin action.

The advantage of the Lantus program is the relatively unwavering flow of basal insulin (a very slight peak may occur 6 to 10 hours after injection of Lantus) and consistent absorption pattern. The disadvantages include the potential for blood sugar rises during the night (due to the lack of a pre-dawn peak) and after dinner (the basal insulin may "wear off" before dinner and take a few hours to reach a stable

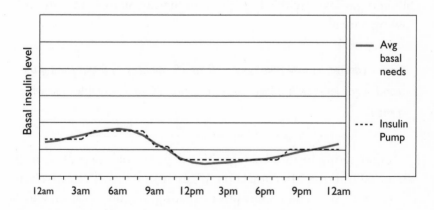

Table 5-5: Basal Option 4: Insulin pump therapy

level following injection). There is also potential for blood sugar drops in the afternoon as the basal insulin level may exceed the liver's production of glucose.

Pump therapy offers the greatest degree of maneuverability in terms of matching basal insulin to the body's needs. Because small pulses of rapid-acting insulin analogs are used to deliver basal insulin, variations in action time are not usually an issue. Pumps also permit temporary changes to basal insulin levels in order to accommodate short-term changes in basal insulin needs (for situations such as illness, high/low activity levels, and stress). Perhaps the greatest drawback to pump therapy is the risk of **ketoacidosis**; any mechanical problem resulting in stoppage of basal insulin delivery can result in a severe insulin deficiency in just a few hours. Without any insulin in the bloodstream, the body's cells begin burning large amounts of fat (instead of sugar) for energy. The result is the production of acidic ketone molecules—a natural waste product of fat metabolism.

Bolus Insulin

Insulin "peaks" are necessary because of the rapid blood sugar rise that occurs after eating carbohydrates (sugars and starches). Carbohydrates usually take about 10 to 15 minutes to begin raising the blood sugar level, with a high point occurring 30 to 90 minutes following a meal.

> *Carbohydrates usually take about 10 to 15 minutes to begin raising the blood sugar level, with a high point occurring 30 to 90 minutes following a meal.*

Rapid-acting insulin analogs (Novolog, Humalog) peak sharply about 60 minutes after injection. These can be used effectively to cover meals when taken just prior to eating. Regular insulin, which peaks 2 to 3 hours after injection, can provide adequate coverage when taken 30 to 60 minutes prior to the meal. However, due to its relatively slow/inconsistent peak and long duration of action (up to six hours), Regular is not usually the preferred insulin to use at mealtimes. In some cases, intermediate-acting insulin (NPH, Lente) is used to cover a meal that will be consumed 4 to 6 hours after injection. For example, NPH or Lente taken at breakfast can be used to cover the carbohydrates eaten at lunch. However, because of their broad and inconsistent peak, NPH and Lente taken in the morning will often cause the blood sugar to drop *before* lunch, followed by a sharp rise after lunch.

A **bolus** *is a dose of fast-acting insulin given to cover the blood sugar rise that occurs soon after eating carbohydrates.*

Table 5-6, below, compares how various insulins "cover" the blood sugar rise that occurs after carbohydrate-containing meals and snacks. As you can see, the insulin analogs (Humalog and Novolog) provide the closest match to the blood sugar rise produced when eating carbohydrates.

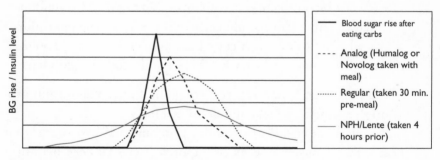

Table 5-6: Insulin coverage after carbs

Putting Them Together

Selecting the best insulin program to meet your needs depends on a number of factors. If you have type 2 diabetes, your pancreas may produce sufficient insulin to meet either your basal or bolus needs, but usually not both. Those with type 2 diabetes can determine their insulin requirements by doing the following:

- Check your blood sugar level at bedtime, have no snack, and then test first thing in the morning. If your blood sugar level rises more than 30 mg/dl (1.7 mmol) while you sleep, your pancreas is not making enough insulin to cover your basal needs; supplementary basal insulin will be required. Lantus is an excellent choice because of its steady, consistent action and relatively low risk for causing hypoglycemia.

- Check your blood sugar before and again 2 hours after eating. If your blood sugar rises by more than 30 mg/dl (1.7 mmol), you will probably need bolus insulin at mealtimes. In most cases, Humalog or Novolog provide the best mealtime insulin coverage. As stated earlier, Humalog and Novolog can be taken just prior to eating. Their rapid peak and short duration of action help to stabilize blood sugar levels after eating. Regular insulin may be appropriate for people with impaired digestion (**gastroparesis**) or when consuming slowly digested foods or large quantities of food at one sitting.

- If your blood sugar is usually over 200 mg/dl (11 mmol), it may be difficult to distinguish between basal and bolus insulin needs. Not to worry: A combination of both basal and bolus insulin should do the trick. Check out the following options.

If you have type 1 diabetes, you are going to need an insulin program that combines basal and bolus insulin.

To select the basal/bolus insulin program that best meets your needs, the "Consumer Reports" approach can be very helpful. I appreciate the way *Consumer Reports* magazine provides objective, side-by-side comparisons of the various features of competitive products. Recognizing that different features are important to different people, this approach makes it easy to choose the products and services that will best meet your individual needs.

Here, then, is my "Consumer's Guide" (Table 5-7) to the most commonly used and recommended basal/bolus insulin programs:

	Overall Control	Work Involved	Hypoglycemia Risk	Lifestyle Flexibility	$ Price
Two Mixed Doses	😞	😊	😞	😞	😊
Morning Mixed w/Evening Split	😐	😊	😞	😞	😊
MDI w/ Bedtime Intermediate	😐	😞	😐	😐	😊
MDI w/ Dinnertime Extended	😐	😞	😐	😐	😊
MDI w/ Basal Insulin	😊	😞	😐	😐	😊
Insulin Pump Therapy	😊	😐	😊	😊	😞

😊 = good   😐 = fair   😞 = poor

Table 5-7: Basal/bolus insulin program comparisons

Option I: Two Mixed Doses
Breakfast: NPH/Lente and Humalog/Novlog
Dinner: NPH/Lente and Humalog/Novlog

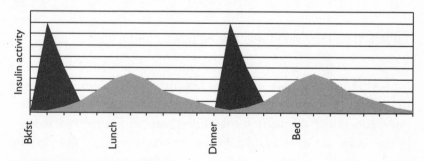

Table 5-8: Two mixed doses

This was a common insulin program used in the 1970s and '80s (with Regular insulin instead of a rapid-acting analog). It is similar to a **premixed insulin** program using two daily injections of 70/30 or 75/25 insulin, except that the proportion of intermediate/fast insulin can be changed when you mix your own doses. With intermediate insulin peaking in the afternoon and at bedtime, this plan limits flexibility in terms of mealtimes/amounts of food. It also predisposes the user to low blood sugars if meals are delayed or exercise added, and to high blood sugars with snacks, larger-than-usual lunches, or delayed injections. The intermediate insulin peak that occurs soon after bedtime is too early for most people, and may cause the blood sugar to drop in the middle of the night and rise in the early morning as the dosage wears off.

Option 2: Morning Mixed with Evening Split
Breakfast: NPH/Lente and Humalog/Novolog
Dinner: Humalog/Novolog
Bedtime: NPH/Lente

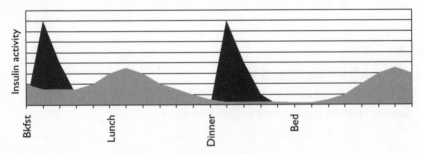

Table 5-9: Morning mixed with evening split

By taking intermediate insulin at bedtime rather than dinner, the peak is shifted to early morning (around the time of the dawn phenomenon, which occurs in most adults) and reduces the risk of lows in the early part of the night. However, the morning intermediate insulin usually results in a blood sugar drop before lunch and a sharp rise after lunch. Afternoon snacks can also be a problem, since the morning intermediate insulin provides minimal coverage in the late afternoon. An additional shot of fast-acting insulin may be needed to cover an afternoon snack.

Option 3: MDI with Bedtime Intermediate
Breakfast: Humalog/Novolog
Lunch: Humalog/Novolog
Dinner: Humalog/Novolog
Snacks: Humalog/Novolog
Bedtime: NPH/Lente

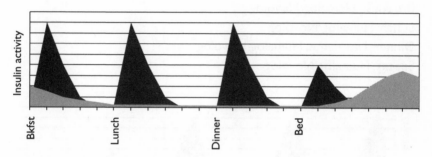

Table 5-10: MDI with bedtime intermediate

Now we enter that zone known as **multiple daily injection** (MDI) therapy. Intermediate insulin taken at bedtime provides an early-morning peak to cover the dawn phenomenon, as well as a pro-longed "tail" of action that ensures the presence of at least a trace of background insulin throughout the day. However, the peak and duration of intermediate-acting insulin can vary from day to day, putting the user at risk for high or low blood sugar in the morning. The relatively low level of basal insulin in the afternoon and evening may result in a blood sugar rise between meals. This type of plan requires an injection of fast-acting insulin at every meal and snack, although snacks that are very low in carbohydrates may not require a shot. Many people find that insulin pens make frequent

Most people on multiple injection programs find that insulin pens are a quick and convenient way to give mealtime and snacktime insulin.

injections less of a chore. Taking fast-acting insulin with each meal and snack offers the freedom to match insulin doses to carbohydrate consumption and activity levels, as well as to make timely corrections for high readings.

Option 4: MDI with Dinnertime Extended

Breakfast: Humalog/Novolog
Lunch: Humalog/Novolog
Dinner: Ultralente, Humalog/Novolog
Snacks: Humalog/Novolog

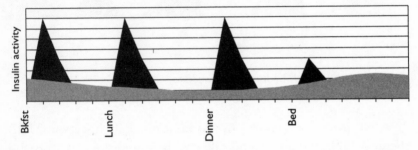

Table 5-11: MDI with dinnertime extended

As with the MDI program described in Option 3, this regimen permits a great deal of flexibility in terms of meals and snacks. Ultralente's modest, prolonged peak can work well for those whose blood sugar varies little during the night. However, it may not provide an adequate peak for those with a pronounced dawn phenomenon. Ultralente's extended duration of action can also present a problem. The prolonged peak can cause blood sugars to drop between meals during the daytime (particularly with exercise). And because Ultralente may work for as long as 36 hours, an overlap can occur when the injections are spaced 24 hours apart. In some instances, two injections of Ultralente, spaced 12 hours apart, are used in an attempt to create a flatter basal insulin profile. However, this rarely achieves the desired effect, as the absorption and action of Ultralente varies considerably from shot to shot.

Option 5: MDI with Basal Insulin
Breakfast: Humalog/Novolog
Lunch: Humalog/Novolog
Dinner: Humalog/Novolog
Snacks: Humalog/Novolog
Any time of day, consistently: Lantus or twice daily (breakfast and dinner) Detemir

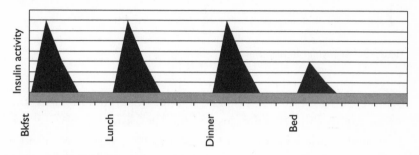

Table 5-12: MDI with basal insulin

Lantus and Detemir are the first insulin formulations that serve as true "basal" insulins. In some individuals, Lantus may show a slight peak 6 to 10 hours after injection, and/or drop off earlier than 24 hours. Detemir must be taken twice daily due to its shorter duration of action (12 to 16 hours). As with any MDI program, injections of fast-acting insulin are necessary with every meal and snack. Lantus must be given in its own syringe (it cannot be mixed with other insulins), meaning that a lot of injections will be necessary. Detemir may be mixed with fast-acting insulin. Although the lack of a "peak" translates into consistent absorption/action from day to day, it can also produce high readings in the morning (as the dawn phenomenon is not adequately covered) or lows in the middle of the day (as basal insulin needs tend to diminish). Still, Lantus and Detemir users tend to experience far fewer lows than those who use intermediate- or long-acting insulin. For those with a pronounced dawn phenomenon, it is reasonable to add a small dose of intermediate-acting insulin at bedtime.

Option 6: Insulin Pump Therapy

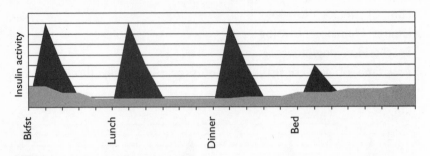

Table 5-13: Insulin pump therapy

Insulin pumps are beeper-sized, battery-operated devices that infuse rapid-acting insulin just below the skin. Pumps are programmed to deliver tiny pulses of insulin every few minutes throughout the day and night (basal insulin), and larger doses at mealtimes (bolus insulin). The insulin is delivered by way of a small, soft plastic tube called an **infusion set**. The infusion set must be changed every couple of days in order to prevent infection and ensure consistent insulin absorption.

The infusion set is usually worn on the abdomen, buttocks, or hip. Most infusion sets feature a "disconnect" mechanism that allows the user to temporarily unhook the pump and tubing for situations such as bathing, contact sports, and intimacy. The pump's tubing is long, strong, and taped in place very securely, so nothing is likely to "pull out" while you sleep or exercise. All pumps are either waterproof or water resistant, so the pump *can* be worn around water if you choose. The pump itself has a secure clip and is usually worn on a belt/waistband or in a pocket. A variety of cases and fashion accessories (Unique Pump Accessories, Pump Wear Inc.) make the pump easy to wear in just about any situation. Pumps also have multiple safety features to ensure against accidental insulin delivery.

One unique aspect of pump therapy is the ability to fine-tune and adjust basal insulin levels throughout the day and night. By matching basal insulin to the liver's normal output of glucose, blood sugars hold steady between meals and during the night. As a result, you can vary your schedule as much as you like in terms of meals, activities, and sleep—in other words, you can live a more normal life. Basal insulin levels can also be adjusted on the fly for events such as menstrual cycles, pregnancy, stress, illness, travel, high-fat meals, and extended exercise.

The ability to fine-tune basal insulin levels at specific times of day and night is a feature unique to insulin pump therapy.

With insulin pumps, mealtime insulin is administered at the touch of a button. The doses are highly precise (some pumps permit dosing in increments as low as twentieths of a unit). Most pumps also offer the option of delivering mealtime boluses all at once or over an extended period of time—in case you expect your meal to take a while to digest.

Benefits of pump therapy include:

1. **Stable blood sugars.** Reductions in HbA1c are common. There are also fewer "high to low" and "low to high" swings.

2. **Fewer low blood sugars.** By using only fast-acting insulin, there is no long-acting insulin peaking at inopportune times. Delayed meals are no longer a problem.

3. **A more flexible lifestyle.** Raise your hand if you can eat, sleep, and exercise at the same times *every* day. The pump lets you choose your own schedule.

4. **Precise dosing** to the nearest half, tenth, or twentieth of a unit; ideal for those who are sensitive to very small insulin doses, such as children and lean adults.

5. **Convenience.** There is no need to draw up syringes every

time you need insulin; just reach to your side and press a few buttons.

6. **No shots.** Multiple daily insulin injections can be uncomfortable and cause skin problems; the pump's infusion set is changed 2 to 3 times a *week*.

7. **No math.** Many pump models can calculate your meal/snacktime boluses for you, based on formulas that you program in.

8. **Easy adjustments for life's little circumstances.** Basal rate changes permit better control during periods of growth, illness, seasonal sports, and menstruation.

9. **Weight Control.** Eat what/when *you* choose; snacks are not required when you use a pump.

10. **Novelty.** Who isn't intrigued by cool graphics, sounds, and buttons? The "high-techness" of the pump can make your diabetes routine seem less, well, routine.

Potential drawbacks to pump therapy include:

1. **A learning curve.** Don't expect good control right away. It usually takes a few months to adjust to wearing the pump and fine-tune the basal and bolus doses.

2. **Inconvenience.** Wearing the pump and tubing around the clock, even during sleep, can cause entanglements once in a while.

3. **Technical difficulties.** As a mechanical device, pumps are prone to occasional infusion set clogs, battery failures, leaks, and glitches.

4. **Skin problems.** Skin can become irritated from infusion set adhesive, and infections can occur if infusion sets are worn in one place for too long.

5. **Ketosis.** The absence of long-acting insulin with pump use can present a problem if insulin delivery is interrupted for

more than a few hours. Very high blood sugar can occur, and ketones may appear in the bloodstream and urine.

6. **Infusion set changes.** Every couple of days, the pump user must change his/her own infusion set. This 3 to 10 minute procedure involves numerous steps and can be momentarily painful or traumatic for the novice pump user.

Certain skills are needed to use a pump successfully. After all, just about any idiot with insulin-dependent diabetes and a decent insurance policy can go on an insulin pump. But to *succeed* with a pump takes preparation, skill, and follow-through.

The assets I consider most important for those seeking an insulin pump are

- motivation/interest in going on a pump;

- a true state of insulin dependence (type 1 or type 2 with little or no insulin production);

- adequate resources to afford the pump and supplies (via insurance or cash reserves); and

- ability to handle basic button-pushing and infusion set change procedures (this can be done by a guardian if the user is very young or physically/mentally challenged).

Certain skills are essential to make a successful transition to the pump. Ideally, these should be mastered prior to starting on the pump:

- carbohydrate counting (using grams rather than exchanges);

- blood glucose monitoring prior to meals and bedtime ($4 \times$/day as a minimum);

- complete record-keeping (including blood sugars, insulin doses, carb intake, and physical activities);

- self-adjustment of insulin doses (based on blood sugar levels, carb intake, and physical activity); and

- understanding of the basic principles of pump therapy (including basic pump operation, infusion set function, the role of basal rates and boluses).

Successful pump use will also require adequate follow-up and fine-tuning once the pump is initiated. This should include:

- basal rate testing throughout the day (fasting for 8- to 10-hour intervals and testing blood sugars to see if they are holding steady);

- fine-tuning of bolus formulas (based on record-keeping);

- troubleshooting and prevention of emergencies such as **DKA** (diabetic ketoacidosis); and

- use of advanced pump features such as extended boluses and temporary basal rates.

To learn more about pump therapy, contact one of the insulin pump manufacturers listed in the Resources section (Chapter 10, p.199) or ask your physician or diabetes educator. Find out if there are insulin pump support groups in your area. Support group meetings offer an excellent forum for meeting other pumpers and finding out about their personal experiences since starting pump therapy.

Substitution Is Permitted

When selecting an insulin program, don't think of it as a lifelong commitment. Many people switch plans because of changes in their lifestyle, or simply because a particular plan fails to do the job. For example, a number of my patients have tried multiple injection programs only to find that the frequent shots were more than they were willing to endure, so they switched back to a three-shot-a-day plan. Others found that long-acting insulin failed to produce consistent overnight control, so they switched to a pump. I have also worked with a number of pump users who switched back to shots—some temporarily during beach season or sports camp; other permanently, due to a need for mealtime structure or personal vanity issues. Just don't forget that the one constant in life is change. You are *not* locked into any particular plan.

And what if your physician doesn't agree with your choice? Ask why. Perhaps he or she has good arguments that will sway your decision. If not, you might want to look for another doctor. After all, this is *your* diabetes, and you deserve the right to manage it in the manner that suits you best.

6

Basal Insulin Dosing

ONCE YOU HAVE SETTLED on an insulin program, the next order of business is to determine the right doses. Think of yourself as a giant lump of clay that needs to be molded, chiseled, and sculpted into fine art. (My personal self-sculpture is a cross between Rocky Balboa and Bond, James Bond.) Any artistic creation takes time, so be patient. Make one adjustment at a time, evaluate the results, and fine-tune before moving on to another area.

Another truism about fine art: Beauty is in the eye of the beholder. What works for some may not work for others. When looking at typical dosing averages and formulas, use them only as a starting point. Individual needs may . . . no, make that *will* . . . vary.

Let's start with the fine-tuning of basal insulin levels. It is best to fine-tune your basal insulin before the mealtime/bolus insulin, because basal insulin serves as the "foundation" for your entire insulin program. When high or low blood sugars appear, it is difficult to know what to adjust unless the proper basal insulin levels have already been established.

In the last chapter, typical basal insulin profiles for people within different age groups were presented. During a person's growth years (prior to age 21), basal insulin requirements tend to be heightened throughout the night. This is due to the production of hormones (growth hormone and cortisol) that counteract insulin and stimulate the liver to release extra glucose into the bloodstream. Following growth years, the production of these hormones is limited primarily to the predawn hours. The dawn effect, as this is called, results in an increased secretion of sugar in the early morning. Thus, basal insulin in most adults tends to peak during the early morning hours.

> *Remember, the purpose of basal, or background, insulin is to offset the liver's normal secretion of sugar into the bloodstream. Because the liver typically secretes different amounts of sugar at different times of day, basal insulin needs also tend to vary at different times of day.*

Initial Basal Doses for Those Injecting Insulin

If you are just getting started with a basal/bolus insulin program, you should start with a conservative dose and increase gradually until your blood sugar levels are within an acceptable range.

The body's insulin requirements are affected by a number of factors, including body size, overall activity level, stage of growth, and the amount of endogenous (internal) insulin production from your own pancreas. To find out how much insulin your pancreas is producing, a blood test called a "**C-peptide**" can be performed. "C-peptide" is a part of the insulin molecule when it is first secreted from the pancreas. Enzymes in the bloodstream break this piece off, leaving two parts: the active insulin molecule, and the C-peptide. C-peptide has no specific function in the body. However, by measuring the amount of C-peptide in the bloodstream, we can determine approximately how much insulin the body is making on its own. A result of less than 0.5 ng/ml indicates that the pancreas is producing abnormally low amounts of insulin.

For those with type 2 diabetes who still produce some of their own insulin, the total daily insulin requirement is usually less than 0.5 units/kg daily. However, this can vary considerably depending on the degree of insulin resistance that exists. A person with insulin-resistant type 2 diabetes who weighs in excess of 250 pounds (113 kg) might require *hundreds* of units of insulin in order to manage blood sugar levels. Another person of similar stature who still produces some of his or her own insulin and is only modestly insulin resistant might require only 10 or 20 units of insulin daily.

For individuals who produce virtually no insulin on their own (including those with type 1 diabetes), insulin requirements are somewhat more predictable. Table 6-1, below, provides typical ranges for total daily insulin needs.

⇓Physical activity⇓ level	Young children	Adolescents	Adults	Older adults
Mostly inactive	0.60–1.2	0.80–2.0	0.60–1.2	0.50–1.0
Moderately active	0.50–1.0	0.75–1.50	0.50–1.0	0.40–0.80
Very active	0.40–0.80	0.60–1.2	0.40–0.80	0.25–0.70

Table 6-1: Daily *total* insulin requirements (units per kilogram body weight)

Recognizing that basal insulin usually accounts for 40–50% of a person's total daily insulin needs (50–60% covering food), basal insulin needs typically fall within the ranges shown in Table 6-2.

⇓Physical activity⇓ level	Young children	Adolescents	Adults	Older adults
Mostly inactive	0.25–0.60	0.30–1.0	0.25–0.60	0.20–0.50
Moderately active	0.20–0.50	0.30–0.75	0.20–0.50	0.15–0.40
Very active	0.15–0.40	0.25–0.60	0.15–0.40	0.10–0.35

Table 6-2: Daily *basal* insulin requirements (units per kilogram body weight)

Translating this to units of insulin, let's take an example:

Debbie is 38 years old and has type 1 diabetes. She weighs 136 pounds, exercises for an hour every day, and has a very active job.

First, we must convert her weight into kilograms (lbs × 0.454 = kg).

$$136 \times .454 = 62$$

Since Debbie is a very active adult, she requires 0.15 to 0.40 units of basal insulin for every kilogram she weighs.

$$62 \times 0.15 = 9.3 \text{ units}$$
$$62 \times 0.4 = 24.8 \text{ units}$$

Debbie is likely to require between 9.3 and 24.8 units of basal insulin daily. Since the "basal/bolus" approach is new to her and she has a history of low blood sugars, she opts to start with 10 units of basal insulin.

Let's take another example. Ben is a teenager with type 1 diabetes who gets a moderate amount of exercise and weighs 105 pounds. He will likely require between 0.30 and 0.70 units of basal insulin per kilogram body weight per day.

His weight in kilograms:

$$105 \times 0.454 = 48$$
$$48 \times 0.30 = 14.4$$
$$48 \times 0.70 = 33.6$$

Having had mostly high blood sugars recently, Ben elects to start with 25 units of basal insulin.

One more example: Jackie is 68 years old and has type 2 diabetes that is poorly controlled on oral medications. It has been determined that her pancreas makes very little insulin. She weighs 210 pounds and hardly gets any exercise.

Her weight in kilograms:

$$210 \times 0.454 = 95$$

She will likely require between 0.20 and 0.50 units of basal insulin per kilogram body weight.

$$95 \times 0.20 = 19$$
$$95 \times 0.50 = 47.5$$

Given that Jackie is brand-new to insulin, she starts with a dose of 20 units of basal insulin.

Fine-Tuning Basal Doses

When injecting basal insulin, our major objective is to establish a dose that maintains steady blood sugar levels through the night (or while sleeping, for those who work night shifts). Ideally, the doses of Lantus or Ultralente, and the nighttime doses of NPH or Lente or Detemir, should produce no more than a 30 mg/dl (1.7 mmol) change while sleeping—assuming that no food is eaten and no heavy exercise is performed before going to sleep.

Basal insulin taken by injection should keep the blood sugar level fairly steady while you sleep.

A consistent rise or drop of more than 30 mg/dl (1.7 mmol) indicates a need to change the basal insulin dosage.

To determine whether or not your overnight basal insulin dose is set correctly, follow this procedure:

- Have a fairly healthy dinner (not too much fat; avoid restaurant and take-out food). High-fat food will cause a prolonged blood sugar rise and will contaminate the test results. Take your usual doses of dinnertime and nighttime insulin.

- If you normally exercise in the evening, go ahead and do so, but keep the intensity and duration modest. Very heavy exercise may cause the blood sugar to drop several hours later, which would also contaminate the test results.

- At least 3 hours after dinner, perform a bedtime blood sugar check. As long as your blood sugar level is above 80 mg/dl (4.4 mmol) and below 250 (13.9 mmol), do not take any food or rapid-acting insulin and proceed with the test. If you are below 80 (4.4), take a snack and try the test another night. If you are above 250 (13.9), give a corrective dose of insulin and try again another night.

- Check your blood sugar again in the middle of the night (or the middle of your sleep time) and first thing in the morning (upon waking up). The middle-of-the-night reading is needed to rule out a potential **Somogyi Phenomenon** (see next page).

If your blood sugar remains within 30 mg/dl (1.7 mmol) from bedtime to wake-up time, your basal dose is probably okay. If it is rising more than 30 mg/dl (1.7 mmol), increase your basal insulin dose by 10% and repeat the test. If it is dropping by more than 30 mg/dl (1.7 mmol), decrease your basal insulin by 10% and repeat the test. Continue adjusting and repeating the test until your blood sugar holds reasonably steady through the night.

For example, if your bedtime reading was 185 mg/dl (9.2 mmol) and your wake-up reading was 122 mg/dl (6.8 mmol), your basal insulin dose is too high since the blood sugar dropped by 63 mg/dl (2.4 mmol) while you slept. Had your bedtime blood sugar been closer to normal, you would have experienced hypoglycemia during the night. Reduce the basal insulin dose by 10%, and run the test again the following night.

Had it risen from 87 mg/dl (4.8 mmol) to 160 mg/dl (8.9 mmol)— a rise of 73 (4.1)—an increase in the basal insulin would be in order.

If your bedtime reading was 95 mg/dl (5.3 mmol) and you woke up at 77 mg/dl (4.3 mmol), the basal insulin dose would not need to be adjusted, because the blood sugar changed by only 18 mg/dl, or 1 mmol, during the night.

Attack of the Killer Somogyi

What about that pain-in-the-neck reading you took during the night? Nobody likes having their sleep interrupted (unless, of course, your hot partner is looking for some action). So that extra reading had better be worth it. Believe me, it is.

In many instances, a blood sugar drop during the night— particularly to levels below 70 mg/dl (3.9 mmol)—causes the body to secrete hormones that raise the blood sugar level by morning, all without your knowledge. This occurrence, known in the medical community as the "Somogyi Phenomenon" (after its discoverer), can interfere with basal dosing decisions if it goes undetected.

Consider the following examples, shown in Table 6-3 and discussed below.

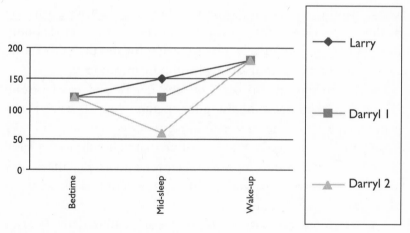

Table 6-3: The Somogyi Phenomenon

Larry, Darryl 1, and Darryl 2 each start and finish with the same blood sugars, indicating a rise during the night. Without knowing the blood sugar in the middle of the night, our first instinct would be to increase the basal insulin for all three. Larry, as it ends up, is experiencing a steady rise throughout the night. An increase in his basal insulin is certainly in order.

However, Darryl 1 experiences a rise, but primarily during the pre-dawn hours. Increasing his dose of nighttime intermediate insulin by 10% (or adding a few units of nighttime intermediate insulin, if he is taking Lantus, Detemir, or Ultralente) would work best.

Darryl 2 is experiencing a Somogyi Phenomenon. He is dropping low in the middle of the night and rebounding to a higher level by morning. Increasing his basal insulin would make the problem worse, not better. A *reduction* in his basal dose by 10%, or possibly adding a bedtime snack, would make the most sense.

Initial Basal Doses for Insulin Pump Users

Basal insulin delivered by an insulin pump comes in the form of tiny pulses of rapid-acting insulin throughout the day and night. Rapid-acting insulin tends to work more efficiently than longer-acting insulin; there is less "waste" involved. As a result, the average pump user requires approximately 20% less basal insulin than those who take intermediate- or long-acting insulin by injection.

I prefer to start pump users on one flat rate of basal insulin delivery and then fine-tune using the methodology described later in this chapter. Of course, it is unlikely that one flat rate will adequately meet your needs. But to assume that you will need a basal "peak" at a certain time of day based on your injection pattern may be completely erroneous and could cause severe low blood sugar when starting on the pump.

To determine an initial rate of basal insulin delivery, two methods are available: the formula methods (which provide a rough approximation) and the empirical approach (which provides a closer approximation).

One of the formula methods is based on your current insulin injection program:

- Add up all the units of insulin you take in an average day by injections, including basal and bolus insulin.

- Divide the total in half (assuming that 50% of your insulin is covering your basal needs).

- Multiply by 0.8 (to take away 20% of the total dose).

- Divide by 24 (to figure the hourly rate).

For example, Marley takes three injections daily (before going on the pump):

Breakfast: 18 NPH and 5 units Novolog (on average)
Dinner: 8 units Novolog (on average)
Bedtime: 12 units NPH

Marley's total insulin for the day is 43 units.
Half that amount is 21.5 units.
Taking away 20% leaves 17.2 units.
Dividing by 24 hours, we get 0.7 units per hour.
Another "formula" calculation is based on body weight. This method should be used by anyone going directly onto the pump without ever having taken insulin injections.

- Take your weight in pounds (to convert kilograms to pounds, multiply by 2.2).

- Divide by 10.

- Divide by 24 (to figure the hourly rate).

If Paul weighs 195 lbs (88.5 kg), we divide 195 by 10 to get 19.5, and divide this by 24 to get 0.8 units per hour.

A more precise method for determining starting basal insulin doses on the pump involves taking your current insulin program, breaking it down into "basal" and "bolus" insulin, and then taking the basal total to figure your hourly rate. Once the injected basal insulin is determined, I would still take away 20% when figuring the initial basal requirements on the pump.

Using Marley's insulin program as an example (see above), I would figure that none of her Novolog doses are used as basal insulin. Since she does not take any insulin at lunchtime, I would figure that approximately 50% of her morning NPH serves as basal insulin (the remainder covering lunch and daytime snacks), and 75% of her nighttime NPH serves as basal insulin (the remainder covering some of her night snack and some of breakfast). Thus, 50% of 18 (9 units) plus 75% of 12 (9 units) are being used as basal insulin, for a total of 18. I would then take 20% away to come up with 14.4, and divide by 24 to come up with an initial rate of 0.6 units per hour.

For someone taking long-acting or basal insulin, I would simply take 20% away from the Ultralente, Lantus, or Detemir dose and divide by 24 to come up with an hourly basal rate.

For example, if Sara is on the following program:

Breakfast: 8 units Humalog (on average)
Lunch: 6 units Humalog (on average)
Afternoon snack: 3 units Humalog (on average)
Dinner: 8 units Humalog (on average)
Bedtime: 2 units Humalog (on average), 25 units Lantus

I would ignore the Humalog doses completely and figure that the Lantus is the only basal insulin. Taking 20% away, we come up with 20 units. Dividing by 24 hours, we get a starting rate of 0.8 units per hour.

Fine-Tuning Pump Basal Rates

This is where the "power of the pump" can really benefit you. The ability to adjust and fine-tune basal insulin levels at different times of day allows you to build a very solid foundation for your complete diabetes management program. Testing, adjusting, and retesting basal rates can be a bothersome process, but it is well worth the effort.

Remember, the purpose of basal insulin is to match the amount of sugar released by the liver into the bloodstream, thus keeping blood sugar levels steady between meals and while you sleep. The right basal rate is one that keeps your blood sugar at a fairly constant level when you have not eaten or bolused for several hours, and are not exercising. Appropriate basal rates must be established in order to obtain quality blood sugar control and enjoy the flexible lifestyle afforded by the pump.

> *The right basal rate is one that keeps your blood sugar at a fairly constant level when you have not eaten or bolused for several hours, and are not exercising.*

All pumps permit the user to set a multitude of different basal delivery rates throughout the day and night. And most offer the choice of setting more than one complete 24-hour program. This can be useful during periods of heightened insulin need (such as sick days, travel days, or prior to menstruation) or decreased insulin need (such as days filled with physical activity or post-menstruation). Use of alternative basal programs will be discussed in more detail in Chapter 8.

To test your basal insulin level, you will need to wait approximately 4 hours after your last bolus and meal/snack. This will give the carbs time to finish digesting and the bolus time to finish working. The conditions that must be met in order to run a successful basal test are listed below.

No food should be digesting

- You may not eat for at least 4 hours preceding the basal test.

- The meal/snack preceding the basal test should be low in fat (no restaurant food or take-out; these tend to raise blood sugars for many hours).

- Do not eat during the basal test, unless your blood glucose is below 80 (4.4).

- You *may* have water or diet beverages during the test.

- Avoid caffeinated beverages during the basal test (caffeine can cause blood sugars to rise).

No bolus insulin should be working during the basal test

- Do not bolus for at least 4 hours preceding the basal test (6 hours if using Regular insulin).

- Do not bolus during the test, unless your blood glucose rises above 250 (13.9).

Your body should be producing its "normal" amount of glucose

- Do not run the test if you have had a low blood sugar within the previous 4 hours; hypoglycemic episodes tend to result in an oversecretion of sugar by the liver for several hours.

- Do not run the test if you are sick.

- Do not run the test if you are taking a steroid medication, unless it is a medication that you plan to continue taking indefinitely at a steady dose.

- Avoid testing just prior to or at the start of your menstrual cycle.

Allow basal insulin to be delivered uninterrupted

- Do not put the pump into suspend just before or during the test.

- Do not disconnect from the pump just before or during the test.

- Do not change your infusion set just before or during the test.

Maintain your normal level of physical activity

- Do not exercise during the blood sugar–testing phase of your basal test.

- You may perform light/moderate exercise soon after your pretest meal/snack if you normally do so at that time.

- Perform your usual daily activities during the basal test.

Monitor blood glucose levels consistently

- Use the same blood glucose meter throughout the testing.

- Use only your fingertips for testing. "Alternate sites" such as the forearm may not be as precise following meals and activity.

I usually start by testing and fine-tuning the nighttime basal rates. Once the overnight rate is matched to the liver's output of glucose, your morning readings should be close to normal. This will make it easier to test the morning segment. Then move on to the afternoon segment, and finally, the evening segment.

To start the test, follow these steps:

- Check your blood sugar at the start of the chosen time period. Remember, it should be at least four hours since the last bolus of Humalog or Novolog (5–6 hours if using Regular insulin).

- If the blood sugar is above 250 (13.9), bolus for the high blood sugar and cancel the test.

- If below 80 (4.4), eat to bring your blood sugar up and cancel the test.

- If the blood sugar is not too high or too low, proceed with the test.

During a basal test, check your blood sugar level every 1 to 2 hours. Less frequent testing may cause you to miss a temporary blood sugar dip or rise. To supplement your fingerstick blood glucose readings, you might choose to wear a GlucoWatch Biographer (Cygnus Corp) which provides readings every 10 minutes or a Continuous Glucose Monitoring System (Medtronic/MiniMed) which provides readings every 5 minutes.

Basal testing should be set up around the framework of your usual mealtimes and sleep patterns. The schedule shown in Table 6-4 on p.117 can be used as a guide for performing a complete set of basal tests. If your blood sugar drops by more than 30 mg/dl (1.7 mmol) during the test period, the basal rate is probably too high. If it rises by more than 30 mg/dl (1.7 mmol), the rate may be too low. The basal rate should be changed and then retested (the next day, if possible) to determine whether the adjustment produces a steady blood glucose level. Continue to adjust and retest until steady blood glucose levels are obtained.

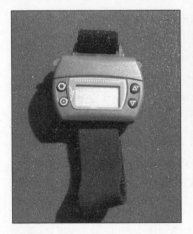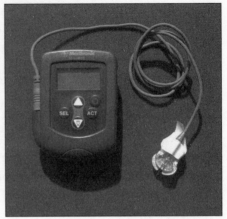

Figure 6-1: Left: The GlucoWatch Biographer (Cygnus Corporation); Right: The Continuous Glucose Monitoring System (Medtronic/MiniMed)

Be aware that any time the blood glucose level is above 180 mg/dl (10 mmol), the kidneys will channel some sugar into the urine. This may produce a slight decrease in the blood sugar concentration. Thus, when performing a basal test with elevated blood sugars, a slight drop-off in the blood sugar is to be expected.

The amount of the change made to basal rates depends on a number of factors, including your current basal levels, the magnitude of the blood sugar changes, and the sensitivity of your pump. Table 6-5 should provide a useful guide.

Basal rates are usually changed one hour prior to the blood sugar changes, since the rapid-acting insulin infused by the pump peaks about an hour later. For example, if your blood sugar rises between 3 a.m. and 7 a.m., you would increase the basal rate between 2 a.m. and 6 a.m. If Regular insulin is used in the pump, the changes should be made 2 hours prior to the blood sugar changes.

It is usually best to maintain a "smooth" basal pattern—one that features just one "peak" and one "valley." Basal patterns that have multiple peaks and valleys throughout the day and night rarely meet the body's needs appropriately.

The following are examples of basal tests and the recommended adjustments for each.

Test	Eat and bolus no later than	Check blood sugar at	Okay to eat and bolus again after
Overnight	7p.m. (eat dinner, then skip evening snacks)	11 p.m., 1 a.m., 3 a.m., 5 a.m., 7 a.m.	7 a.m.
Morning	3 a.m. (have a bedtime snack, then skip breakfast and morning snack)	7 a.m., 9 a.m., 11 a.m., 12 p.m.	12 p.m.
Afternoon	8 a.m. (eat breakfast, then skip morning snack, lunch, and afternoon snacks)	12 p.m, 2 p.m., 4 p.m., 6 p.m.	6 p.m.
Evening	2 p.m. (eat late lunch, then skip afternoon snack and have a late dinner)	6 p.m., 8 p.m., 10 p.m., 11 p.m.	11 p.m.

Table 6-4: Sample schedule for basal tests

Blood sugar change during test		Current basal level (units/hr)		
		0.0–0.35	0.4–1.0	>1.0
	Modest (30–100 mg/dl; 1.7–5.6 mmol)	0.05 (if pump allows) or 0.1	0.1	0.2
	Large (>100 mg/dl; >5.6 mmol)	0.1	0.2	0.3

Table 6-5: Change to basal rates

- **Christine** recently started using a pump and is using a flat basal rate of 1.2 units per hour throughout the day and night. To verify her overnight basal rate, she had a low-fat dinner at 6 p.m., and nothing else to eat the rest of the night. Her blood sugars during the test were as follows:

10 p.m.: 117
12 a.m.: 187
2 a.m.: 238
4 a.m.: 240
6 a.m.: 218

Christine's blood glucose level rose sharply between 10 p.m. and 2 a.m., then held steady from 2 a.m. until 6 a.m. (the slight drop-off from 4 to 6 a.m. is likely due to the loss of sugar through the urine). I would recommend that she increase her basal rate by 0.3 units per hour (to 1.5) from 9 p.m. until 1 a.m., and repeat the testing (taking readings just until 2 a.m.) Her basal rate from 1 a.m. until 5 a.m. appears to match her liver's output of glucose since the blood sugar level remained fairly constant from 2 a.m. to 6 a.m.

- **Bret**'s basal rates are 0.20 units per hour from 6 a.m. until 9 a.m., and 0.15 units per hour the rest of the day. To confirm his morning basal rate, his parents had him skip breakfast and test his blood sugars through the morning. The results were as follows:

7 a.m.: 184
8 a.m.: 192
9 a.m.: 177
10 a.m.: 190
11 a.m.: 224
12 p.m.: 259

Bret's blood sugars held steady from 7 a.m. to 10 a.m., so the

0.2 basal from 6 a.m. to 9 a.m. looks good. The blood sugar rise from 10 a.m. to noon requires a basal increase to 0.20 from 9 a.m. to 11 a.m. Bret's parents should plan to test his midday basal rates next, with breakfast at 6 a.m., and blood sugar tests from 10 a.m. until 2 or 3 p.m.

- **Gina** is currently using basal rates of:

0.5 units/hr 12 a.m.–7 a.m.
0.4 units/hr 7 a.m.–1 p.m.
0.3 units/hr 1 p.m.–8 p.m.
0.4 units/hr 8 p.m.–12 a.m.

To verify her overnight basal rates, Gina had dinner at 7 and nothing else the rest of the night. Her blood sugars during the test were as follows:

11 p.m.: 158 mg/dl
1 a.m.: 146 mg/dl
3 a.m.: 144 mg/dl
5 a.m.: 97 mg/dl
7 a.m.: 77 mg/dl

Gina's blood glucose levels remained fairly constant from 11 p.m. until 3 a.m., verifying her basal rates from 10 p.m. to 2 a.m. However, the level dropped significantly from 3 a.m. until 6 a.m. A standard adjustment would call for a 0.1-unit reduction in her basal settings from 2 a.m. until 6 a.m. However, this would create a very "choppy" basal pattern, with peaks at midnight to 2 a.m. and again at 6 to 7 a.m. Instead, I would recommend lowering the basal to 0.4 from 2 a.m. all the way until 7 a.m., and would then repeat the basal test with a snack permitted at 11 p.m. and readings taken at 3 a.m., 5 a.m., and 7 a.m.

Obviously, fine-tuning basal insulin levels can become complex.

This is a great opportunity to reach into your "tool chest" and pull out that member of your health care team who specializes in this sort of thing—most likely your CDE or pump trainer. You are the ultimate decision-maker regarding your diabetes plan, but it never hurts to seek out an expert opinion!

7

Bolus Calculations

AHH . . . PIZZA HOT FROM the oven. The aroma of fresh-popped popcorn. Cold Italian ice on a hot summer day. That mysteriously tasty cream center in Oreo cookies.

Basal insulin would meet our needs just fine . . . if we never ate. But we do eat, and eating makes blood sugars rise. So for the above, and countless other, culinary delights, we have something called **bolus insulin**.

Boluses are doses of insulin given to cover the blood sugar rise produced by the carbohydrates in our meals and snacks. Boluses are also used to lower blood sugars that are higher than we want. Boluses can be adjusted based on a myriad of factors, especially our level of physical activity before and after eating. There are many other secondary factors that influence bolus requirements; these will be presented in the next chapter. For our purposes here, in most instances, most boluses are based on the following:

1. the amount of carbohydrate in the meal or snack

2. the blood sugar level at the time of the meal or snack

3. the amount of planned (or completed) physical activity

For those of you who are mathematically inclined (you know who

> *In most instances, boluses are based on carbohydrates to be eaten, blood sugar levels, and physical activity.*

you are—your checkbooks actually balance each month, and if they don't, it's the bank's mistake), boluses are typically calculated as follows:

Bolus = (Insulin to cover carbs + insulin to correct blood sugar
      level) × adjustment for exercise

Let's take a look at each of these main components one at a time.

1. Insulin to cover carbs

As is the case with basal insulin, appropriate bolus insulin dosing requires a great deal of fine- tuning. What we are looking to develop is called an "**insulin-to-carb (I:C) ratio**." In other words, we need to determine how many grams of carbohydrate are covered by each unit of rapid-acting insulin. For example, a 1 to 10 ratio means that one unit of insulin covers 10 grams of carbohydrate. A ratio of 1 to 20 means that each unit covers 20 grams. Calculating the food bolus is easy when you know your I:C ratio. Simply divide your carbs by your ratio. If each unit covers 10g and you consume 65 grams, you will need 6.5 units of insulin (65/10 = 6.5).

Note that using a I:C ratio of 1:10 will mean giving larger boluses than if you use a ratio of 1:15. A 30g snack will require 3 units if you're using a 1:10 ratio, but only 2 units if you're using 1:15. As the second number in the ratio goes up, the amount of insulin goes down.

The beauty of an I:C ratio is that it gives you the flexibility to eat as much or as little carbohydrate as you choose while still maintaining control of your blood sugars. However, it is common to require different I:C ratios at different times of day. This is due to

changes in hormone levels (which affect insulin sensitivity), physical activity (which enhance insulin sensitivity), and the amount of
basal insulin overlapping with the bolus.

Two methods exist for determining initial I:C ratios. Whichever
method you choose, it might be best to be conservative. During the

---

It is common to require different I:C ratios at different meals and snacks.

---

adjustment process, it is better to run a few high readings than to
run the risk of a severe low.

The 500 Rule

The 500 rule is based on an assumption that the average person
consumes (via meals and snacks) and produces (via the liver)
approximately 500 grams of carbohydrate daily. By dividing 500 by
your average number of units of insulin daily (basal *plus* bolus), you
should get a reasonable approximation of your I:C ratio.

Avg. Units Insulin Daily (basal + bolus)	Approx. I:C Ratio
8–11	1:50
12–14	1:40
15–18	1:30
19–21	1:25
22–27	1:20
28–35	1:15
36–45	1:12
46–55	1:10
56–65	1:8
66–80	1:6
81–120	1:5
>120	1:4

Table 7-1: Bolus calculation using the 500 rule

For example, if you take a total of 25 units of insulin in a typical day, each unit of insulin should cover approximately 20 grams of carbohydrate (500/25 = 20). If you take 60 units daily, your I:C ratio would be 1 unit per 8 grams of carb (500/60 ≅ 8).

The obvious weakness to this approach is that it assumes that all people eat about the same amount of food and produce the same amount of glucose. Those who are heavy or tend to eat relatively large amounts of carbohydrate will underestimate their insulin requirement with this approach; those who are lean or eat relatively little will overestimate their requirement.

The Weight Method

This approach is based on the fact that insulin sensitivity diminishes as body mass increases; hence each unit of insulin will cover less food in a heavier person than in a lighter person.

One of the potential problems with this system is that it fails to consider body *composition*. An individual who weighs 250 pounds but is very muscular will be much more sensitive to insulin than a person of similar weight who has a great deal of body fat. Another problem is that this system fails to consider stages of growth and hormone production. A growing adolescent will require significantly more mealtime insulin than a senior who weighs the same amount.

Weight (lbs)	Weight (kg)	Approx. I:C Ratio
<60	<27	1:30
60–80	27–36	1:25
81–100	37–45	1:20
101–120	46–54	1:18
121–140	55–64	1:15
141–170	65–77	1:12
171–200	78–91	1:10
201–230	92–104	1:8
231–270	105–123	1:6
>270	>123	1:5

Table 7-2: Bolus calculation using the weight method

Fine-Tuning and Verifying I:C Ratios

Remember, it is best to establish your basal insulin levels before attempting to fine-tune your boluses. Any basal insulin changes made after fine-tuning your boluses will require additional bolus adjustments.

Fine-tuning boluses is best done empirically (what my people call "trial and error"). You will want to verify the I:C ratio at each meal and snack separately, because insulin sensitivity changes throughout the day.

Keep detailed written records when testing your I:C ratios. It is best to eliminate factors other than food that might be affecting the results of the tests. For example, do not include data collected during or after strenuous exercise, unless you exercise strenuously on a daily basis at a consistent time of day. Also, don't count readings during an illness or major emotional stress, at the start of a menstrual cycle, or after a low blood sugar. Meals with very high fat content or unknown carb content (such as heavy restaurant meals) should not be included in your analysis.

To analyze your data, take a look at your blood sugar level before the meal and then again at least 3 hours later (to give the insulin a chance to finish working) with no other food, unusual exercise, or boluses in between. Because strange things can happen on any given day, I like to consider 1 to 2 weeks of data when coming to a decision regarding the I:C ratio.

For example, consider the following data:

Date	Pre-breakfast blood sugar in mg/dl (mmol)	Carbs (grams)	Bolus insulin (units)	Pre-lunch blood sugar in mg/dl (mmol)	Conclusion
6/1	175 (9.7)	50	6.5	101 (5.6)	1:8 makes BS drop
6/2	83 (4.6)	50	4.0	78 (4.3)	1:12 held BS steady
6/3	62 (3.4)	75	5.0	226 (12.5)	Don't count—low to start
6/4	151 (8.4)	50	6.0	93 (5.2)	1:8 makes BS drop
6/5	210 (11.6)	40	6.0	113 (6.3)	1:7 makes BS drop a lot
6/6	75 (4.2)	75	5.0	180 (10.0)	1:15 makes BS rise
6/7	123 (6.8)	50	5.0	86 (4.7)	1:10 makes BS drop a bit
6/8	99 (5.5)	90	7.0	52 (2.8)	1:14 makes BS drop ???
6/9	97 (5.4)	30	2.5	114 (6.3)	1:12 held BS steady
6/10	154 (8.5)	65	3.0	274 (15.2)	1:20 makes BS rise a lot

Table 7-3: Analyzing a 10-day record

Based on this information, I would be tempted to assign an I:C ratio of 1 unit per 12 grams of carb. I would throw out the data on 6/3 due to the low reading prior to breakfast. I would also throw out the data on 6/8—it is inconsistent with every other result, and the meal was much larger than usual (perhaps it was a Denny's Grand Slam breakfast). The data indicates that an I:C ratio of greater than 1:12 produces a blood sugar rise; less than 1:12 produces a drop. When used, 1:12 held the blood sugar fairly steady—the lunch readings were within 30 mg/dl of the breakfast readings.

Fine-tuning I:C formulas can be a challenging proposition, even for the most highly trained and experienced health professional. The more detailed you keep your records, the better. You might discover subtle influences from a variety of factors.

For example, one of my patients, Betty, had high readings every Sunday at lunchtime, but normal readings the rest of the week. The reason? Most likely, church. Betty is very passionate about prayer. In addition to sitting still for several hours, the adrenaline surge she gets from prayer is consistently producing a blood sugar rise. The solution: Use her usual 1:10 formula during the week, but increase to 1:6 on Sundays.

Another patient, Gerry, was experiencing very inconsistent blood sugars prior to dinner despite having a consistent lunch and using a consistent 1:15 bolus formula at lunchtime. In reviewing his records, we found that most of his dinnertime lows were preceded by morning workouts; most of his dinnertime highs followed no morning workout. The solution: Use a 1:10 formula at lunch after sedentary mornings, but decrease to 1:20 following morning exercise.

Given the complexities of determining bolus formulas, it is worthwhile to have a second set of eyes look over your records. Don't hesitate to ask a loved one or close friend to help you form a conclusion; even an "untrained" eye can be helpful in detecting patterns. Then have your physician or diabetes educator review your data, to confirm that your conclusion is a reasonable one.

2. Insulin to correct blood sugar

The second part of "bolus by numbers" focuses on fixing blood sugars that are either too high or too low. Assuming that your blood sugar levels are going to vary, it will be necessary to make adjustments to your meal and snack boluses, in order to get your readings closer to your target by the next time you test. This is referred to as "**correction insulin**" or, in some cases, "sliding scale insulin."

To understand this approach, imagine that you are a famous archer from Sherwood Forest, trying to win Maid Marian's hand by winning an archery contest. As you focus on your goal (the target, not Maid Marian), what do you aim for? Dead center, of course! If you aim toward the sides or edges of the target, your chances of a bull's-eye are greatly diminished. In fact, you might miss the target completely, resulting in a chorus of laughter from the evil Sheriff's luxury suite.

Remember, blood sugar control is far from an exact science. The goal is to have blood sugar levels that are within a desirable *range* most of the time. To do so, always aim for the center of that target. If your target range is 70 (3.8) to 170 (9.4), aim for 120 (6.7). If your range is 80 (4.4) to 200 (11.1), aim for 140 (7.8). That way, you increase your chances of landing within the target range at your next reading.

For example, if you designate your "target" blood sugar to be 120 mg/dl (6.7 mmol) and your pre-meal reading happens to be 175 (9.7 mmol), you will need to add "correction" insulin to your meal dose. Does this guarantee that you will be on target at your next reading? No, but it sure increases the odds that you will be. If you don't add any correction insulin, it's like aiming to be too high again next time. In archery terms, it's like aiming for the outer edge of the target instead of at the center.

Likewise, if your blood sugar is 80 (4.4 mmol), you will need to take some insulin away from your meal dose. This increases your chances that the blood sugar will rise a bit and let you hit the target range by the next meal. If you don't reduce your meal dose when your blood sugar is below your target, you increase your chances of missing the target completely and experiencing a low blood sugar before the next meal.

To figure out how much insulin to add or subtract based on

the pre-meal blood sugar level, three pieces of information are needed:

1. Your current (*pre*-meal or wake-up/fasting) blood sugar level. Testing your blood sugar after eating is not of much value, since the reading will be affected by what you just ate.

2. Your target blood sugar. A specific number is needed— ideally, near the midpoint in your target range.

3. Your **sensitivity factor.** This has nothing to do with how good a listener you are or your willingness to miss a football game for the sake of shopping. Your sensitivity factor is how much each unit of insulin lowers your blood sugar.

> *The more you weigh and the more insulin you take, the less every unit will lower your blood sugar.*

Each person's sensitivity to insulin is unique. In general, the heavier you are and the more insulin you take, the less sensitive you will be to each individual unit. A number of approaches can be used to determine your sensitivity factor, but one method tends to work best: Call it the "1,500/1,800 rule." Here is how it works:

Figure your average total daily insulin, including basal and bolus insulin. Then divide it into both 1,500 and 1,800. The result is an approximate range (in mg/dl) of how much one unit of insulin will lower your blood sugar (see Table 7-4). To convert to mmol, divide by 18.

When choosing an initial sensitivity factor, most people take a nice "round" number. For instance, if you're using 80 units a day, you might choose 20 mg/dl (or 1.2 mmol) as your sensitivity factor. If you're using 40 units a day, you might choose 40 mg/dl (2.2 mmol).

If you want to be aggressive about bringing down high readings, choose a sensitivity factor toward the low end of your range. That way, you will take a bit more insulin to bring down a high reading. If you are making a concerted effort to prevent low blood sugars, choose a correction toward the high end of your range. That will have you taking a bit less to bring down high readings.

Average Total Daily Insulin (all basal + all boluses)	Sensitivity Factor (mg/dl)— how much 1 unit lowers blood sugar	Sensitivity Factor (mmol)— how much 1 unit lowers blood sugar
5 units	300–360	17–20
7 units	200–250	11–14
10 units	150–180	8.3–10
12 units	125–150	6.9–8.3
15 units	100–120	5.6–6.7
18 units	80–100	4.4–5.6
20 units	75–90	4.2–5.0
25 units	60–72	3.3–4.0
30 units	50–60	2.8–3.3
35 units	43–51	2.4–2.8
40 units	38–45	2.1–2.5
45 units	33–40	1.8–2.2
50 units	30–36	1.67–2.0
60 units	25–30	1.39–1.67
70 units	21–26	1.17–1.44
80 units	19–23	1.06–1.28
90 units	17–20	0.94–1.11
100 units	15–18	0.83–1.00
120 units	12–15	0.67–0.83
140 units	11–13	0.61–0.72
160 units	9–11	0.50–0.61
180 units	8–10	0.44–0.56
200 units	7–9	0.39–0.50

Table 7-4: Sensitivity to insulin based on daily insulin usage

Examples

If Dave takes an average of 28 units of insulin daily, we get

1,500 / 28 = 54
1,800 / 28 = 64

This means that every unit of insulin should lower Dave's blood sugar approximately 54–64 mg/dl. To simplify the calculation, we round off to 60.

If Dave's target blood sugar is 100 (5.6), he would add 1 full unit for every 60 points over 100 and subtract 1 unit for every 60 points below 100. Expressed as a formula, his correction is:

(Current blood sugar − 100) / 60

If Dave's blood sugar is 222, we get (222 − 100) / 60, or 2.0 units. He needs 2.0 extra units to "correct" his blood sugar down to 100. If he needs 3 units for his meal, he would increase the dose to 5.

If his blood sugar is 76, we get (76 − 100) / 60, or −0.4 units. He needs to *take away* 0.4 units (or approximately ½ unit) from his meal dose. If he needs 3 units for his meal, he would decrease it to 2.6 (or 2.5).

Let's look at another example. April takes a total of 75 units of insulin daily. Each unit should lower her blood sugar 20 (1,500 / 75) to 24 (1,800 / 75) mg/dl. Because April's blood sugars are typically high and she has not experienced any severe low blood sugars, she chooses to be aggressive and assume that each unit lowers her by 20 mg/dl. This will have her taking more correction insulin for highs than if she assumed a 24-point drop per unit.

If April's target blood sugar is 120, she will add 1 full unit for every 20 points over 120, and subtract 1 unit for every 20 points below 120. Her correction formula is:

(Current blood sugar − 120) / 20

If April's blood sugar is 161, she will need (161 − 120) / 20, or 2 units, in addition to the insulin she gives to cover her food. If her blood sugar is 310, she will need (310 − 120) / 20, or 9 ½ extra units.

Correction Factors May Vary

Just as insulin-to-carb formulas can vary from meal to meal, correction formulas may also vary. Don't be surprised if each unit of insulin lowers your blood sugar much more at night than during the day. In the evening, many people experience a drop-off in hormones that counteract insulin. As a result, each unit of insulin can lower the blood sugar more at bedtime as compared to breakfast, lunch, and dinner.

> *For many people, each unit of insulin lowers the blood sugar more at night than during the day.*

In my own case, each unit of insulin lowers my blood sugar consistently by 40 mg/dl when given at breakfast, lunch, or dinner. However, each unit lowers me by 60 mg/dl when given at bedtime. My bedtime correction formula is (BS − 120) / 60 rather than (BS − 120) / 40.

Sensitivity factors may also change over time. With weight gain, most people lose some sensitivity to insulin, and the sensitivity factor tends to decrease. Changes in physical activity levels can also affect insulin sensitivity. Prolonged periods of inactivity due to illness, injury, travel, or sedentary occupations may lower insulin sensitivity and require a reduction in the sensitivity factor. Long-term increases in activity can produce the opposite effect.

Verifying Your Sensitivity Factor

You can verify the accuracy of your sensitivity factor empirically by doing the following:

1. Test your blood sugar at least 4 hours after your most recent bolus of rapid-acting insulin (6 hours if using Regular insulin).

2. If the blood sugar is elevated, apply your correction formula and give the appropriate dose of insulin. Go about your usual activities, but do not eat or exercise for the next several hours.

3. Test your blood sugar 4 hours later.

4. Calculate your blood sugar drop and divide by the number of units you gave. This should come close to your correction factor. If it does not, repeat the process the next day. If the results are similar to those from the first day, adjust your correction factor accordingly.

For instance, yesterday I checked my blood sugar 4 hours after lunch, and it was 205 mg/dl (darned hoagie!). Applying my daytime formula of (BS − 120) / 40, I gave 2.1 units. Before dinner, my blood sugar was down to 112. I dropped 93 points (205 − 112). Dividing by 2.1 units, I come up with 44 points per unit—not exactly 40, but close enough!

Beware of unused insulin

Patience is a virtue. Unfortunately, we all know someone who never abides by that philosophy. They want everything right away. No time to mess with something that isn't working. Fix it. Change it. Replace it. *Immediately.*

Sometimes, things work themselves out—if given a chance. Take insulin, for example. The fastest insulin still takes about 4 hours to complete its job. Four hours. Not 10 minutes. Not 1 hour. Not even 2 hours. Blood sugar levels taken 1 or 2 hours after a bolus will usually still be elevated because the insulin has not finished working. At that point, you have two choices: Blast away at the elevated blood sugar with a fully loaded correction bolus, or sit back and wait to see what happens.

For those who want to be aggressive about their control but not thrust into repeated hypoglycemic seizures, the best option lies somewhere in the middle. The "unused insulin rule" lets us figure whether or not we need additional insulin based on what is still left working from a previous bolus.

The unused insulin rule is based on typical absorption patterns seen with rapid-acting insulin. Keep in mind that insulin absorption and action can vary from person to person and from situation to situation. I have seen cases where Humalog and Novolog seem to be spent in just over 2 hours, and other instances where the insulin seems to continue working for as long as 5 or 6 hours. In *most* cases, the actions of Humalog and Novolog follow the pattern shown in Tables 7-5 and 7-6.

For example, if you gave yourself 6 units for a 3 p.m. snack, then check your blood sugar at 5 p.m., you still have 30% of your bolus remaining; 6 units × 30% = 1.8 units (or 2 units, if rounding off).

Time since bolus was given:	½ hour	1 hour	1½ hrs	2 hrs	2½ hrs	3 hrs	3½ hrs	4 hrs
Insulin "used up"	10%	30%	50%	70%	80%	90%	95%	100%
Insulin remaining	90%	70%	50%	30%	20%	10%	5%	0%

Table 7-5: Unused insulin

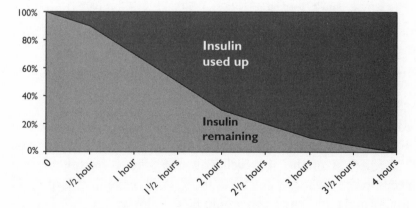

Time since bolus

Table 7-6: Unused insulin

If you gave 12 units at dinner and check your blood sugar 3 hours later, you still have approximately 1.2 units (12 × 10%) remaining.

For the sake of simplicity, some people choose to assume that one-third of their insulin is "used up" each hour, as shown in Table 7-7.

Time since bolus was given:	I hour	2 hours	3 hours
Insulin "used up"	33%	67%	100%
Insulin remaining	67%	33%	0%

Table 7-7: Aggressive calculation of unused insulin

Those who want to be more conservative (i.e., give less insulin to cover highs) assume that 25% is used up each hour, as shown in Table 7-8.

Time since bolus was given:	I hour	2 hours	3 hours	4 hours
Insulin "used up"	25%	50%	75%	100%
Insulin remaining	75%	50%	25%	0%

Table 7-8: A conservative calculation of unused insulin

Although these approaches tend to be less precise than the one shown in Table 7-5 on page 133, they make for easier calculations on the run.

Regardless of the approach you use, your correction insulin needs to be reduced by any bolus insulin still remaining. Expressed as a formula, the correction would be as follows:

(normal correction insulin) − (insulin remaining from previous bolus)
= safe dose to cover a high blood sugar

If you would normally take 4 units to cover a high reading, but 3 units are still remaining from an earlier bolus, it would be wise to give only 1 unit. If you would normally take 2 units for a high reading but 2.5 units are still active, you should not take any correction insulin. In fact, if the "insulin remaining" exceeds your usual correction factor by a great deal, you might need to snack in order to prevent a low blood sugar in the next couple of hours.

For those using Regular insulin, the typical action curve is shown in Tables 7-9 and 7-10.

Time since bolus was given:	1 hour	2 hrs	3 hrs	4 hrs	5 hrs	6 hrs
Insulin "used up"	10%	30%	60%	80%	95%	100%
Insulin remaining	90%	70%	40%	20%	5%	0%

Table 7-9: Unused insulin, using Regular insulin

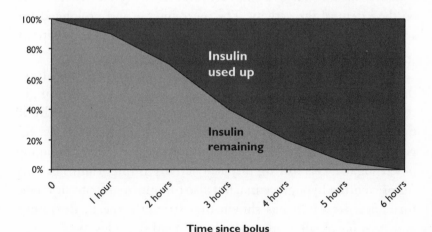

Time since bolus

Table 7-10: Unused insulin, using Regular insulin

3. Adjustment for exercise

Okay, let's see what we have so far. Bolus insulin is calculated based on the amount of carbohydrate and the blood sugar level. Put the food insulin together with the correction insulin and we have our grand total. Right? Well, not exactly.

You see, a unit of insulin is not always a unit of insulin. Let me put that another way. A unit of insulin given in one situation may not act the way a unit acts in another situation. The single most important factor in determining daily variations in insulin's potency is physical activity. Not just exercise, but any form of physical activity—including yardwork, cleaning, shopping, filing, sex, playing in the dirt, and anything else that has us using our muscles more than usual.

> *Physical activity can make muscle cells more sensitive to insulin for many hours, depending on the duration and intensity of the activity.*

Muscles are one of the main targets for insulin. With increased workload, muscle cells become much more sensitive to insulin. This enhanced insulin sensitivity may continue for many hours, depending on the extent of the activity. The more intense and prolonged the activity, the longer and greater the enhancement in insulin sensitivity is going to be.

With enhanced insulin sensitivity, insulin exerts a greater force than usual. A unit that usually covers 10 grams of carb might cover 15 or 20. A unit that normally lowers the blood sugar by 50 mg/dl might lower it by 75. Thus, the need to adjust boluses for pending, and in some cases previous, physical activity. Managing blood sugar levels during physical activity is important not only for preventing hypoglycemia, but also for improving physical performance: Research has shown that strength, speed, flexibility, and stamina are all hindered by high blood sugar levels.

Some forms of physical activity, most notably high-intensity/short duration exercises and competitive sports, can produce a short-term rise in blood sugar levels followed by a delayed drop. This is due primarily to an adrenaline surge. Adjustment for these types of activity will be discussed later in this chapter.

Aerobic (Cardiovascular) Activities

Most daily activities and aerobic exercises (exercises performed at a sub-maximal level over a period of 20 minutes or more) will have a tendency to cause blood sugar levels to drop, due to enhanced insulin sensitivity and accelerated sugar metabolism. To prevent low blood sugar, you can reduce your insulin dose, increase your food intake, or both.

When exercise is going to be performed within an hour or 2 after a meal, the best approach is usually to reduce the meal-time bolus. Because both aspects of the bolus (the food part and the blood sugar correction part) are influenced by physical activity, both need to be reduced. To accomplish this, I like to use an activity "multiplier." Essentially, this means that you calculate your mealtime bolus as usual (based on the food and the blood sugar level), and then multiply the bolus by a factor that results in a lower dose as shown in Table 7-11.

Activity multipliers	Short duration (15–30 minutes)	Moderate duration (40–60 minutes)	Long duration (>60 minutes)
Low intensity (RPE 8–11)	0.90	0.80	0.70
Moderate intensity (RPE 12–15)	0.75	0.67	0.50
High intensity (RPE 16–18)	0.67	0.50	0.33

Table 7-11: Calculating bolus with activity

Rating of Perceived Exertion (RPE) Scale	
6	
7	Very, very light*
8	
9	Very light
10	
11	Fairly light
12	
13	Somewhat hard
14	
15	Hard
16	
17	Very hard
18	
19	Very, very hard*
20	

* Note that very, very light activities constitute little more than resting and typically do not require any insulin adjustments. Very, very hard activities are usually "anaerobic"—they cannot be performed for more than a few minutes and tend to cause a short-term rise in blood sugar levels.

Table 7-12: Rating of Perceived Exertion (RPE) Scale

Exercise multipliers are based primarily on the duration and intensity of the activity. While duration is fairly easy to measure, intensity is, shall we say, in the eye of the beholder. The "Rating of Perceived Exertion" chart above (see Table 7-12) is a simple yet accurate means of assessing the intensity of your workout. It takes into account the speed/pace of the activity, your current physical condition, number/size of muscles utilized, your skill/familiarity with the activity, and the workout environment.

For example, if Mindy is planning a leisurely 20-minute bike ride after dinner (she considers it "fairly light"), she would multiply her dinner bolus by 0.90, which would effectively reduce her dose by 10%. If she plans a much more intense 60-minute ride up and down hills (which she considers "very hard"), she would multiply her dinner dose by 0.50, which would reduce her dose by 50%.

With improved physical conditioning, exercise will tend to produce less of a blood sugar drop. A smaller reduction in the usual insulin dose will be needed.

Over time, most people experience a "conditioning effect." This means that we tend to become more efficient at performing the same activity once we have had a chance to practice it. As a result, we burn less fuel and may require less of an insulin reduction. This also holds true for those who use food to prevent lows during exercise—less food is required to maintain the blood sugar level as we become better conditioned.

When exercise is going to be performed before or between meals, reducing the bolus at the previous meal would only serve to drive the pre-workout blood sugar very high. A better approach would be to take the normal bolus at the previous meal, and then snack prior to exercising.

The amount of the snack depends once again on the duration and intensity of the workout. The harder and longer your muscles are working, the more carbohydrate you will need to eat, in order to maintain your blood sugar level. It is also based on your body size: The bigger you are, the more fuel you will burn while exercising, and the more carbohydrate you will need.

Exercising after meals is better for those trying to lose weight—you don't need to consume any extra food, and cutting back on insulin promotes the loss of body fat.

Granted, there is no way of knowing exactly how much you will need, but the carb amounts listed in Appendix D should serve as a safe starting point. It is based on the typical number of calories burned during different forms of exercise, the proportion of calories derived from sugar versus fat (with higher-intensity exercises, we tend to burn a higher proportion of calories from carbs rather than fat), and the extent to which counter-regulatory hormone production raises the blood sugar level during the activity.

To use the chart, find your approximate body weight and look down the list to find an activity similar to what you will be doing. The number in the column represents the grams of carbohydrate that you will need per hour of activity. If you will be exercising for half an hour, take half the amount listed before participating in the activity. If you will be exercising for 2 hours, take the full amount before you begin, and take it again 1 hour into the workout.

For example, someone who weighs about 200 pounds (91 kg) and swims at a slow pace for 30 minutes would need to consume 24–30 g of carbohydrate before swimming, to keep his or her blood sugar level steady. Note that this is half of the amount required for a full hour.

If someone weighing about 150 pounds (68 kg) plans to do 45 minutes of housework, he or she should take 7–15 g carb, which is 75% of the 1-hour amount.

Someone who weighs 125 pounds (57 kg) and is going to play baseball for 2 hours should plan to consume 17–25 g carb before the first hour and another 17–25 g before the second hour. This amount represents the midway point between recommendations for 100 pounds (45 kg) and 150 pounds (68 kg).

Of course, the best way to fine-tune your snack supplement for exercise is to test your blood sugar before and after the activity. If it holds steady, you have found the magical carb value. If it is rising, cut back on the number of carbs. If it is dropping, add some more next time. For activities lasting several hours, check your blood sugar hourly to determine whether your carb requirements change during the course of the activity. Frequent testing is also a good way to "touch up" high or low readings, by adjusting the amount of carb at your next hourly snack.

As mentioned earlier, you should also watch for a conditioning effect. Less carb may be needed to hold your blood sugar steady as you become more familiar with your activity and more physically fit.

For those of you who use insulin pumps and choose to lower basal insulin for extended periods of physical activity, the amount of carbohydrate you will need (or the frequency with which you need to eat) will be diminished. More about this will be presented in the next chapter.

Anaerobic Exercise and Competitive Sports

As mentioned previously, it is not unusual to experience a blood sugar rise at the onset of high-intensity/short-duration exercise and competitive sports. This is caused by a surge of adrenaline, which counteracts the effects of insulin and stimulates the liver to release extra sugar into the bloodstream. Exercises that often produce a short-term blood sugar rise include:

- Weight lifting (particularly when using high weight and low reps);

- Sports that involve intermittent "bursts" of activity, like baseball or golf;

- Sprints in events such as running, swimming, and rowing;

- Events where performance is being judged, such as gymnastics or figure skating; and

- Sporting events in which winning is the primary objective.

If you notice that your blood sugar rises consistently during these types of activities, it is in your best interest to take extra insulin beforehand. Case in point: One of my teenage patients always saw his blood sugars rise well into the 300s (17–22 mmol) every time he had a hockey game. During practices, his blood sugar would drop steadily. But games caused just the opposite effect. Once he started taking extra insulin before games, his blood sugars stayed closer to normal, and his performance went up a notch. In his first tournament trying this approach, he won his first-ever MVP trophy!

To determine how much insulin to take before a high-intensity event, first consider how much your blood sugar normally rises during the course of an event. If it rises 200 mg/dl (5.6 mmol) and your sensitivity factor is 50 (2.8) points per unit, you will need to give 4 units about half an hour beforehand. If you normally rise 70 mg/dl (3.9 mmol) and your sensitivity factor is 30, you will need a little more than 2 units half an hour beforehand.

If you are nervous about giving insulin before exercise, check your blood sugar more often than usual (perhaps every half hour), and have glucose tablets or some other form of fast-acting carbohydrate nearby. Or, you might choose to give half the insulin you are supposed to give, and adjust the amount based on your control during and after the event.

Delayed Effects

Ever finish a workout with a terrific blood sugar level, only to go low overnight or the next morning? As it turns out, many aerobic activities (particularly those that are long or intense) and most anaerobic exercises cause blood sugars to drop several hours later. There are two reasons why this takes place.

First, following heavy exercise, the body's muscle cells become highly sensitive to insulin. This results in lower-than-normal blood sugars if the usual insulin doses are given. Though it is possible for increased insulin sensitivity to last for several days, it most commonly lasts for 8 to 12 hours. Second, muscle cells tend to become depleted of **glycogen** (sugar stores) during intense exercise. For the next several hours, muscles draw extra sugar from the bloodstream to replenish these stores, resulting in an even greater blood sugar drop. When this occurs, it is called **delayed-onset hypoglycemia**.

Great. It has a name. So did the plague. What exactly can be done about it?

The best way to deal with delayed-onset hypoglycemia is to document it and then make adjustments to prevent it. By documenting it, I mean keeping good, detailed records to find out when your delayed drop takes place. It might be after only certain types of activities, or only a specific number of hours later. For example, I have found that my blood sugar drops before lunch the day after I play full-court basketball. Not half-court basketball. Not one-on-one or "rough house" (an organized form of hog-the-ball). Only full-court seems to do it. And it only seems to affect me the following morning—not overnight.

It took a series of mid-morning lows before it dawned on me exactly what was going on. Now I reduce my breakfast bolus by about 50% the morning after full-court basketball, and the problem has gone away.

I have had many patients whose blood sugars drop during the night following heavy exercise during the day. Options for managing this type of problem include:

- lowering the basal insulin during the night (which is easy to accomplish if using an insulin pump or taking NPH or Lente at bedtime);

- having an extra snack at bedtime; or

- reducing the bolus usually given to cover carbs and high blood sugar at bedtime.

Managing Pre-Activity Highs

It is not usually dangerous to exercise with a high blood sugar level, as long as there is at least a basal level of insulin in your body. Without a minimum level of insulin, exercise will cause the blood sugar to rise further and may accelerate the production of **ketones**—acidic by-products of fat metabolism. If ketones build up in large amounts, they can alter the delicate pH balance in the bloodstream and body tissues and produce a life-threatening condition called **diabetic ketoacidosis** (DKA).

> *It is generally not dangerous to exercise with a high blood sugar level, as long as there is at least a basal level of insulin in your body.*

If your pre-exercise blood sugar is inexplicably high, there is one way to make sure you have sufficient insulin to allow for a safe exercise session: Check your urine (or your blood) for ketones. The presence of small, moderate, or large ketones in the urine indicates a lack of insulin in the body. Do not exercise if you have ketones in your urine. Instead, drink plenty of water and contact your physician immediately.

If you do not have ketones or your blood sugar is just moderately elevated, it should be safe to exercise. However, high blood sugars during exercise can be a problem for anyone who wants to maximize his or her performance. As mentioned in Chapter 3, optimizing blood sugar levels during exercise can enhance your strength, speed, stamina, flexibility, and mental concentration—all of which add up to better athletic performance. (See Table 7-14.)

To adjust for high blood sugar prior to exercise, it is best to obtain a reading approximately 30 minutes before the activity. This will give the bolus insulin time to kick in before you start your activity. Because exercise has a tendency to amplify insulin's effects, I recommend a bolus that is half of what you would normally give to cover a high reading. For instance, if your normal sensitivity factor is 40 points per unit, assume an 80-point drop per unit if you are about to exercise. If possible, test your blood sugar during and after your workout, to see how well this works, and adjust as needed the next time around.

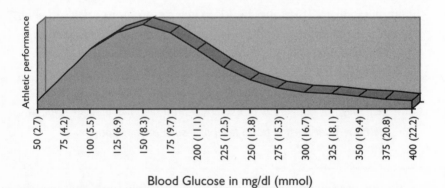

Table 7-14: Exercise performance

Inactivity: Sensitivity in Reverse

What goes up, must come down. Just as increased physical activity causes improvements in insulin sensitivity, decreased activity can have just the opposite effect.

Anyone who has gone from an active job to a sedentary job knows what this is all about. It also happens when we spend hour after hour sitting in planes, trains, or automobiles. Those who are recovering from surgeries or injuries tend to go through it, as well. We call it "insulin resistance," or simply a reduced sensitivity to insulin. And it requires increases in your usual insulin doses just to get the same job done.

There are two ways to handle this problem. One would be to get up off your butt and start moving. If that is not possible (or just not in your immediate plans), consider taking your bolus doses up in small increments—perhaps using a bolus multiplier of 1.1 , then 1.2, then 1.3, and so on, until your pre-meal readings are back within your target range.

Bolus Timing

Let's see . . . so far, the bolus is based on three dimensions: the food part (using the I:C ratio), the blood sugar part (using a correction formula), and the activity part (employing a multiplier for after-meal exercise). Three dimensions should just about do it. Unless, of course, you live in the real world—where the fourth dimension, time, is of the essence.

The timing of your boluses can make or break their effectiveness. Boluses given too early can cause low blood sugar followed by high readings several hours later. Boluses given too late can produce significant hyperglycemia soon after eating. A properly timed bolus, in the proper quantity . . . now, there's a thing of beauty.

The first and only assumption is that you will be using a rapid-acting analog (Humalog or Novolog) for your boluses. If you are still using Regular insulin, take all the advice given below and back everything up by 20 to 30 minutes. The timing of your boluses should be based on a few key variables: the type of food you will be eating, your pre-meal blood sugar level, and the presence or absence of impaired digestion.

Glycemic Index

Glycemic Index (GI) refers to the rapidity with which food raises the blood sugar level. Although virtually all carbohydrates convert into blood sugar eventually, some forms do so much faster than others. Pure glucose is given a GI score of 100; everything else is compared to the digestion/absorption rate of glucose. See Appendix B for a GI list for many common foods.

> *Glycemic Index (GI) indicates the speed with which food raises the blood sugar level.*

Most starchy foods have a relatively high GI; they digest easily and convert into blood sugar quickly. Likewise, foods that have glucose or dextrose in them tend to have a high GI. Table sugar (sucrose) has a moderate GI, while fructose (fruit sugar) and lactose (milk sugar) are slower to raise blood sugar. Foods that contain fiber or large amounts of fat tend to have lower GIs than comparable foods that do not. For example, french fries tend to raise the blood sugar more slowly than baked potatoes. Apples tend to do it a bit more slowly than apple juice.

Foods with a high GI (greater than 70) tend to raise blood sugar the fastest, with a significant "peak" occurring in 30 to 45 minutes. Examples include bread, potatoes, cereal, and rice. For these types of foods, it is best to bolus 15 to 30 minutes prior to eating. This will allow the insulin peak to coincide as closely as possible with the blood sugar peak. And that, of course, will produce the best possible after-meal control. Bolusing for high-GI foods just before or after eating would produce a significant after-meal blood sugar "spike," because the insulin would lag behind the blood sugar rise by about half an hour.

Foods with a moderate GI (approximately 40–70) digest a bit slower, resulting in a more modest blood sugar peak approximately 1 hour after eating. Examples include ice cream, orange juice, cake, and carrots. Bolusing 30 minutes before eating these types of foods could produce a low blood sugar soon after eating. It is best to bolus immediately prior to foods with a moderate GI.

Foods with a low GI (below 40) tend to produce a slow, gradual blood sugar rise. The blood sugar "peak" is usually blunted and may take several hours to appear. Examples include pasta, milk, yogurt, beans, and whole fruit. For these types of foods, bolusing prior to eating tends to produce a blood sugar drop soon after eating, followed by a marked blood sugar rise a few hours later as the food takes effect and the insulin wears off. For these types of foods, a few bolus options are available:

- Bolus 10 to 15 minutes after eating. This usually gives the food enough of a head start before the insulin kicks in.

- Split the bolus into two or three parts, each given about an hour apart starting at the mealtime. Wearing a watch with an alarm can help remind you to give the after-meal boluses.

- Take Regular insulin with the meal, rather than a rapid-acting insulin analog. With its delayed peak and prolonged action, Regular insulin does a better job of matching the blood sugar rise from low-GI foods.

- If you use an insulin pump, extend the bolus delivery over an hour or two.

In summary:

High-GI food:	Bolus before eating
Moderate-GI food:	Bolus while eating
Low-GI food:	Bolus after eating

Blood Sugar

The second major variable to affect the timing of your boluses is the pre-meal blood sugar level. To avoid an after-meal blood sugar drop or spike, it is best to give the bolus earlier (when the blood sugar is elevated), and later (when the blood sugar is below your target). Table 7-15, below, combines the glycemic index and pre-meal blood sugar to determine optimal bolus timing.

Bolus timing in relation to meal	High-GI food	Moderate-GI food	Low-GI food
BG above target range	30–60 min. prior	15–30 min. prior	0–5 min. prior
BG within target range	15–30 min. prior	0–5 min. prior	10–15 min. after
BG below target range	0–5 min. prior	10–15 min. after	30–45 min. after

Table 7-15: Optimal bolus timing

When Will It Digest?

Another factor that will influence the timing of your boluses is the rate at which your digestive system operates. **Gastroparesis** is a form of neuropathy (nerve disease) that affects thousands of people with diabetes. Those who suffer from gastroparesis tend to digest food very slowly, as the stomach is too sluggish to empty food into the intestines where it can then be absorbed into the bloodstream. People with gastroparesis may benefit from using Regular insulin rather than a rapid-acting analog, an extended bolus (if using an insulin pump), or simply bolusing 15 to 30 minutes after eating whenever symptoms are present.

Digestion can also be affected by nausea. Anyone who is prone to vomiting after meals, including those with flu-like symptoms, women suffering from morning sickness, and patients receiving chemo or radiation therapy should wait a reasonable length of time after eating to make sure the food will "stay down" before giving a bolus.

A similar issue can be had by finicky eaters. Young children, for example, may not always eat what is presented to them. My kids tend to go through phases where they would rather play with their food than eat it, followed by phases where they'll eat every food item in the house, including the box it came in.

If you are dealing with an unpredictable/inconsistent eater, you can replace uneaten carbs with caloric beverages like juice. However, it might be more practical to "pick your battles" and just save the boluses for immediately after meals and snacks.

8

Adjusting to
the Real World

THERE YOU ARE. ARMED with the ideal basal insulin program to meet your body's background insulin needs and bolus equations that would impress your high school algebra teacher. Off you go to conquer your favorite Italian restaurant.

There's going to be a half hour wait for a table. "No problem," you say to yourself. "My basal insulin should take care of me." Well, that 30-minute wait turns into 60 minutes, thanks to a huge party that just won't leave. Irritated, you start walking past the table, clearing your throat as loudly as possible. No movement. Time to hit the bar.

As time ticks away, the Diet Cokes turn into gin and gingers. *Finally,* the hostess calls out your name (mispronounced, but close enough). Elation turns once again into frustration as she leads your group to the smoking section. "I asked specifically for non-smoking," you tell her.

"Are you sure? Well, I'll have to see what we have available."

Fifteen minutes later, your group finds its way to a table in non-smoking. Your frustration grows once again as you check your blood sugar to find that it has risen a great deal since you left home. "I haven't eaten a thing . . . How could this happen?" you ask yourself.

Oh well, nothing a little extra insulin can't fix. Your meal features the usual array of breadsticks, salads with rich dressings, pastas with heavy cream sauces, and cheesecake for dessert. Counting your carbs as carefully as possible, you bolus the exact amount as dictated by your bolus formulas. You even give the insulin after your meal because it contains a lot of slow-digesting foods. A plan that can't possibly fail, right?

Wrong. On the way out of the restaurant, you start feeling a bit dizzy and confused. No problem—you whip out your trusty meter, dab on a drop of blood, and it reads . . . LOW. Now you're really confused. How could you possibly be low after a meal like that? No matter, grab a handful of mints from the hostess stand (it's the least they could do after making you wait so long!) and let someone else drive home.

Hopefully, all is not lost. You *did* count your carbs and bolus the right amount, so your bedtime reading should be decent. In fact, it is just a little bit on the high side, but given all you had to eat, that's not so bad. A minor insulin touch-up, and it's off to bed.

That night, you have a nightmare about a giant lasagna chasing you down, trying to turn you into a late-night snack. To make matters worse, you have to get up several times during the night to go to the bathroom. Upon waking the next morning, you discover that your blood sugar is way up. "That's it," you tell yourself. "I'm never going to that restaurant again. From now on, nothing but good old trusty American fare."

Welcome to the "real world." Things don't always go as planned, and blood sugars don't always turn out as predicted.

In Chapter 3, I presented many of the factors that influence blood sugar levels. So far, we have focused on the "primary" factors: carbohydrates, physical activity, and the body's endogenous (internal) production of sugar. Now it's time to discuss the secondary factors: those pesky things that tend to mess with good control.

Secondary Factors that Tend to Raise Blood Sugars

Anxiety/Stress

Anxious moments abound in most of our lives. From speaking in public to test-taking to a simple visit to the doctor or dentist, many events elicit a stress hormone response that causes, among other things, a sharp blood sugar rise. Of course, different events cause different responses in different people. What causes a great deal of anxiety for you might have no effect on someone else. The key is to look for patterns: a consistent blood sugar response in a given situation. It may be helpful to record the possible causes of your high blood sugars on your written records, and then tally the causes to determine whether specific situations account for a large number of high readings. One of my patients did just this and found that high blood sugars were occurring consistently on Tuesday and Thursday evenings following phone calls from her daughter (who happened to be going through an ugly divorce). Obviously, thinking about and discussing the divorce was causing her a great deal of blood sugar–raising anxiety.

> *The first step in making intelligent adjustments is identifying patterns of high or low readings in a given situation.*

The Adjustment:

Many anxious moments occur spontaneously. However, some can be predicted. If you notice a consistent pattern of high blood sugars with certain events, consider giving yourself a small dose of rapid-acting insulin an hour or two prior to the event. This will accommodate for the stress hormones produced in anticipation of the event as well as during the event itself. The first time you try the adjustment, be certain to check your blood sugar frequently to see how well the extra insulin is working. A student I work with tends to run very high blood sugars when taking standardized tests in school. Her parents agreed to give her extra insulin at breakfast on the mornings of standardized testing, and her blood sugar turned out to be very close to normal at lunchtime. Who knows? Keeping your blood sugar near normal might help you to do a better job of coping with the event itself.

Caffeine

A natural stimulant, caffeine tends to cause a rise in blood sugar levels approximately 1 hour after ingestion. It does this by stimulating the secretion of stress hormones and promoting the breakdown of fat (rather than sugar) for energy. Granted, the amount of caffeine found in most foods is insignificant. However, consumption of large amounts of caffeine at one time can produce a noticeable blood sugar rise. Below is a list of some of the major sources of caffeine:

Stay-awake pills:	100–200 mg
Brewed coffee (8 oz):	100–120 mg
Espresso:	100 mg
Instant coffee (8 oz):	60–80 mg
Tea (8 oz):	30–50 mg
Cola (12 oz):	30–45 mg
Cold tablets:	30 mg
Chocolate bar:	20–30 mg
Chocolate milk (12 oz):	10 mg

The Adjustment:
If you suspect that caffeine may be causing your blood sugar to rise, either look for a lower-caffeine substitute or take a little extra rapid-acting insulin when consuming high-caffeine foods/beverages. To determine the amount of insulin you need, test your blood sugar and then consume the caffeinated item with no other food (bolus only for the carbs in the caffeinated item). Check your blood sugar again in 3 hours. Divide the rise by your sensitivity factor. For example, one of my patients has a 16-ounce black coffee each morning and finds that

her blood sugar rises by about 80 mg/dl (4.4 mmol). Since each unit of rapid insulin lowers her by 40 mg/dl (2.2 mmol), she needs to take 2 units of insulin just to offset the effects of the caffeinated coffee on her blood sugar.

Disease Progression

Most people with type 1 diabetes go through a "honeymoon" phase soon after diagnosis: For several weeks, months, or even years, the pancreas continues to produce a small amount of insulin. This results in blood glucose levels that are stable and near normal, particularly overnight and first thing in the morning. As the pancreas loses the ability to produce insulin, blood sugars become higher and more erratic. Likewise, type 2 diabetes becomes progressively more difficult to manage, as the body becomes more insulin-resistant and the pancreas loses the ability to produce sufficient amounts of insulin to control blood sugar levels.

The Adjustment:

For those with type 1 diabetes who are exiting the "honeymoon," fasting (or morning) blood sugars will tend to be elevated—perhaps for the first time. Increases in basal insulin are usually needed to manage overnight blood sugar levels. Bolus increases may also become necessary, as the pancreas loses the ability to produce basal insulin throughout the day. For those with type 2 diabetes, the gradual loss of insulin-producing beta cells means that insulin dosage requirements will gradually increase. Whenever blood sugars come in above target for three days in a row, it is time to increase the insulin dose at the preceding meal (or the basal insulin dose, if the high readings are occurring first thing in the morning).

Fatty Foods

Consumption of large amounts of fat in a meal or snack can cause blood sugar levels to rise in a gradual manner over a period of 6 to 10 hours or more. This delayed rise is in addition to the immediate rise caused by carbohydrates. The exact mechanism by which fat causes a delayed rise in the blood sugar is not entirely understood, but it is believed to be a combination of (1) partial conversion of fatty acids into glucose; (2) insulin resistance caused by elevated fatty acids in the bloodstream; and (3) a slowdown in the digestion of some carbohydrates consumed along with the fat.

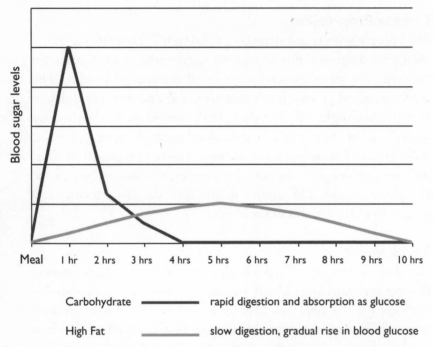

Table 8-1: Glucose rise after consuming food

Although there is no specific amount of fat that causes a delayed blood sugar rise in every person, having more than 20 grams of fat in a meal or snack certainly increases the likelihood that it will occur. Some foods commonly associated with high fat content and delayed blood sugar rises are listed below.

- **Restaurant foods:** Meals prepared at restaurants usually have a great deal of fat added during preparation.

- **Take-out food:** pizza = 10–20 g fat per slice; hot wings = 2–3 g each; Chinese food: egg roll = 15 g, fried rice = 13 g/cup, sweet and sour pork = 25 g/cup

- **Fast food:** small cheeseburger = 15 g fat; Big Mac = 30 g; average taco = 11 g; sausage/egg/cheese sandwich = 40 g

- **Fried foods:** oils used in preparing fried food contain 10–15 g fat *per tablespoon*; fried fish sandwich = 23 g; fried chicken patty = 14 g; small order of french fries =15 g

- **High-Fat meats:** most cuts of beef, lamb, pork, dark meat chicken/turkey, and sardines contain approximately 8–15 g fat per 3 ounces (a deck-of-cards-sized serving); ground round/hamburger = 20 g; ribs and sausage = 25 g; most lunch meats = 10 g per slice; a hot dog = 15 g

- **Cheesy dishes:** approximately 70% of cheese is pure fat; American/cheddar/Swiss cheese = 8–10 g per ounce (or slice); mozzarella/parmesan = 6–7 g per ounce

- **Dessert items:** an average slice of chocolate cake = 15 g fat; ice cream = 10–15 g per half-cup; a cinnamon bun = 25 g; 1 doughnut, muffin, slice of cake, or chocolate bar = 10–20 g; 1 slice apple pie or cheesecake = 20 g

- **Salty snacks:** chips = 10 g fat per handful; peanuts = 10–15 g per small handful; a medium movie theater popcorn = 60 g fat (*without* butter topping); nachos with cheese = 20–30 g

You will need to determine (based on your own experience) how much fat is required to produce a delayed blood sugar rise. For example, I find that a single slice of pizza rarely causes my blood sugar to rise after the first couple of hours. However, after eating two or more slices, I usually see a significant rise over the next 6 to 8 hours.

The Adjustment:
When a delayed rise in blood glucose is anticipated, two options are available. For those taking insulin by injection, *intermediate*-acting insulin (NPH or Lente) tends to do a nice job of offsetting the effects of fat. Taking a small dose of intermediate insulin along with your rapid-acting mealtime insulin provides a nice one-two

punch: The rapid insulin covers the immediate rise produced by the carbohydrates, and the intermediate insulin covers the delayed rise produced by the fat.

The amount of intermediate insulin will vary depending on the type of meal and amount of fat you are consuming. As a starting point, try taking a dose equivalent to 5–10% of your total insulin for the entire day. For example, if you average a total of 50 units of insulin for the day (basal + bolus combined), give yourself 2½ to 5 units of NPH or Lente with a high-fat meal.

> *The delayed blood sugar rise caused by high-fat foods can be offset with a small dose of intermediate insulin or a temporary basal increase.*

If you are using an insulin pump, the adjustment is much simpler. A temporary basal increase lasting approximately 8 hours should do the trick. Start with an increase of 50–60% above your usual basal insulin level, and see if your blood sugar holds steady over the next 10 to 12 hours. If your pump allows you to make basal adjustments in percentages, the change should be easy. If your pump only allows you to set one flat rate for a temporary basal change, you will need to do the math by hand. For example, if your basal rates are normally 0.7–0.8 following your high-fat meal, increase to 1.2.

Growth and Weight Gain

During a young person's growth years, insulin needs rise steadily, due to increases in the production of sex and growth hormones (which counteract insulin and stimulate additional glucose production by the liver) as well as increases in body size. The accumulation of body fat also increases insulin requirements by causing insulin resistance.

The Adjustment:

All aspects of the insulin program will need to change with significant gain (or loss) of weight. Adjustments should be made in proportion to the amount of weight gained or lost. With a 10% change in body mass, changes are usually needed in basal insulin levels, insulin:carb formulas, and the sensitivity factor. For example, a person who goes from 120 to 135 pounds (57–64 kg) and has blood sugars that are usually above his or her target range should increase basal, bolus, *and* correction insulin by approximately 10%. Someone who goes from 240 to 215 pounds (114–102 kg) and experiences repeated low blood sugars should *reduce* his or her doses by 10%.

Illness/Infection

Infections are common in people with diabetes, particularly when blood sugar levels are chronically high. Infection-fighting white blood cells do not work well when the blood sugar is elevated. Extra glucose in the bloodstream also provides nourishment for viruses and bacteria (aiding and abetting the enemy!). Infections, in turn, cause the body to produce stress hormones that drive the blood sugar even higher and make insulin less effective.

Infections commonly affect the respiratory system, urinary tract, and skin. Symptoms include:

- Chronically high blood sugars

- Fever

- Nausea

- Dehydration

- Enlarged glands

- Thick yellow, green, or milky secretions

Ketones may be present in the urine during an illness. This is caused by insulin's lack of effectiveness (as a result of all the stress hormones that are being produced). It is important to check your blood sugar and ketones frequently during an illness and stay in close contact with your health care team.

The Adjustment:

Even without your usual food intake, be sure to keep taking your basal insulin during an illness. Without basal insulin, your blood sugar will go dangerously high and you will put yourself at risk of diabetic ketoacidosis (DKA). When in DKA, your blood has become so acidic that you will likely be vomiting and extremely achy. Treatment for DKA requires an immediate trip to your nearest emergency room.

In most cases, extra basal insulin is required during an illness. If your blood sugars are repeatedly high and you are not spilling ketones in your urine, consider increasing your basal insulin by 25%. If you have small or moderate ketones, increase by 50%. Large ketones: Increase by 75–100%. The basal insulin increase is in addition to your usual bolus doses, including correction doses to cover high blood sugars.

Keep in mind that insulin will not absorb properly into the bloodstream if you are not adequately hydrated. It is essential to drink plenty of fluids during an illness—preferably clear, caffeine-free fluids. Most adults should consume 1 cup per hour while awake; small children should consume ½ cup per hour.

Rebounds from Lows/Somogyi Phenomenon

High readings that follow hypoglycemic episodes may be caused by a **rebound effect**. Significant low blood sugars (particularly those that elicit symptoms such as shaking and sweating) usually result in the production of adrenal hormones that raise the blood sugar and inhibit insulin's action for the next several hours. This causes the blood sugar level to be unusually high several hours later and makes it difficult to bring down with your usual dose of correction insulin.

When low blood sugars occur during sleep, it is common for the body's own natural "rebound" to kick in and produce high readings upon waking. This is referred to as a Somogyi Phenomenon. Many people sleep through these mild lows and believe that they need *more* insulin to control the morning highs. Of course, increasing the nighttime insulin would only make the problem worse! The following symptoms may indicate that you are going low and rebounding during the night:

- nighttime sweating

- cool body temperature

- restlessness

- headache/hangover-like symptoms

- rapid heartbeat upon waking

- nightmares

- not feeling well-rested in the morning

It is a good idea to check your blood sugar periodically, at the midpoint of your sleep time, to verify that your blood sugar is not dropping while you sleep. If getting up in the middle of the night doesn't appeal to you, try wearing a GlucoWatch (Cygnus Corp) or Continuous Glucose Monitor (Medtronic/MiniMed) during the night; review the readings the next day (see the Resource list in chapter 10 for contact information).

The Adjustment:
Unfortunately, it is difficult to predict when (or if) a rebound is going to occur after a low blood sugar. If you experience a consistent rebound at a consistent time following lows (or certain types of lows), it is reasonable to give a dose of insulin designed to prevent the rise. For example, if your blood sugar always rebounds to the 300s (17–22 mmol) at bedtime after midday lows, you might consider taking some intermediate-acting insulin (NPH or Lente) after treating the low. If you consistently rebound to very high levels 2 to 3 hours after readings below 40 (2.2), you might consider taking a few units of rapid-acting insulin after you have treated the low.

Speaking of treatment, another way to prevent a significant rebound is to refrain from over-treating the low. Eating excessive amounts of food when you are low is like throwing gasoline on a fire. Proper treatment of lows will be discussed in the next chapter.

Steroids
Steroidal medications such as cortisone and prednisone are used to

treat asthma, arthritis, emphysema, and muscle/joint inflammation. These drugs create insulin resistance and raise blood sugar
levels—sometimes dramatically. Inhalers (containing albuterol)
and topical steroids (in cream or ointment form) can also raise
blood sugar levels. For those using a steroid medication on an
ongoing basis, changes in steroid doses can lead to blood sugars that
are higher or lower than usual.

The Adjustment:
Some steroids are more potent than others, and their onset/duration
of action can vary. Ask your physician about the specific medication
that you plan to use. In most cases, single doses of a steroid medication (for example, an injection for knee or joint inflammation) will
raise the blood sugar for 8 to 72 hours. Basal insulin may need to be
increased by as much as 50–200% until the steroid wears off.

Other Medications
Diuretics, Dilantin, niacin (vitamin B3), epinephrine (for bee
stings), and cough/cold remedies that contain epinephrine all have
a tendency to cause a short-term rise in blood glucose levels. Thyroid medications (taken by those with an underactive thyroid
gland) also induce modest elevation.

The Adjustment:
If you have been taking any of these medications over an extended
period of time, no insulin dosage adjustments should be necessary.
However, if you are starting, stopping, or changing a dosage,
increases in bolus insulin immediately following the medication
may be required. In the case of thyroid medication, changes in
basal insulin may be necessary when starting or changing a dose.

Surgery
Medical procedures, ranging from oral surgery to a cardiac bypass to a
facelift, have certain physiological and psychological consequences.
Among these is a stress response by the body (in response to an invasion
by "foreign fingers") as well as the mind (in anticipation of the event).

There is also a recovery period that involves bed rest and a certain degree of discomfort. What's it all mean for your diabetes? Yep, high blood sugars. And at the worst possible time. A "speedy recovery" hinges on good blood sugar control. The body's tissues heal better and with less risk of infection, when the blood sugar is near normal.

> *Prior to any procedure involving anesthesia, have your diabetes doctor send a letter to your anesthesiologist detailing your pre-op, intra-op, and post-op care.*

The Adjustment:

If your anesthesiologist offers to control your blood sugars for you during and after the procedure, take her up on it. The medical team will monitor your blood sugar frequently and infuse insulin directly into your bloodstream via an IV to keep your blood sugar as close to normal as possible.

For outpatient procedures, you will probably be asked to manage your own diabetes. That's okay—it's not as complicated as it may seem. Since most procedures require you to fast beforehand, surgeons will typically schedule their diabetic patients first thing in the morning (Take advantage of it! We might as well get *something* for having this disease!).

Even though you won't be eating beforehand, you will probably need extra basal insulin to offset the effects of stress hormones prior to and during the procedure, and lack of activity (and discomfort) after the procedure. As is usually the case, bolus insulin should only be given if/when you are going to eat.

Here's a quick guide to help you manage:

If you are using an insulin pump: Stay connected to the pump before during and after the procedure. Raise your basal insulin by 50% an hour or two before the procedure, and continue the temp basal increase until several hours afterwards. Cover your pre-surgery blood sugar with your usual correction bolus, and bolus as usual for your after-surgery meals/snacks.

If you are taking Lantus, Detemir, or Ultralente at any time, or NPH/Lente at night: Take your usual dose of basal insulin. An hour or 2 prior to the procedure, check your blood sugar and administer a correction bolus as needed. After the procedure, check again and bolus as needed.

If you are taking NPH or Lente in the morning: Give 50% of your usual dose of NPH or Lente in the morning. Include Humalog or Novolog to cover any high blood sugars upon waking. Cover all meals during the day (including lunch) with Humalog/Novolog. If you are unable to eat, test your blood sugar every 2 to 3 hours and administer correction insulin as needed.

Travel

Travel can present special challenges for people with diabetes. Due to changes in meals, activity, and schedules, blood sugars may change quite a bit when you travel. Time zone changes can also wreak havoc on control. You should monitor your blood sugar more often when traveling, but be careful when visiting a place where the altitude is much higher than you are used to: Some blood glucose meters do not give accurate readings above a certain altitude (check your owner's manual to see if your meter may be affected).

When in transit, whether it be by plane, train, bus, car, boat, or flying saucer, your blood sugar levels may run higher than usual. This is caused by a combination of factors, including the stress of travel and the fact that prolonged sitting tends to diminish sensitivity to insulin.

The Adjustments:

Plan to take a little extra insulin on travel days. Increase your boluses by 25–50% during trips lasting 2 to 4 hours. For trips that last much longer, consider increasing your basal insulin by about 40%. Look for opportunities to walk around at rest stops, up and down aisles, or on deck. This will help with the circulation and action of your insulin. If you need to take an insulin injection on a plane, only inject half as much air as usual into the vial. Cabin pressure is lower than the air pressure on the ground, so you won't need to build up as much pressure inside the bottle.

When traveling across time zones, some insulin program adjustments may be necessary. Those using insulin pumps should adjust the clock on their pump to correspond with the local time. This will help ensure that basal insulin peaks will correspond to your sleep schedule at your destination.

Those taking Lantus or Detemir may continue on their usual program, making sure to keep the doses 24 or 12 hours apart (respectively). This may mean taking the basal insulin at a different time than you are accustomed to. For example, if you normally take your Lantus at 10 p.m. and travel west across three time zones, you should begin taking it at 7 p.m. (local time) once at your destination. Upon traveling home, you can resume your usual injection time of 10 p.m.

For those who take a basal insulin that "peaks" (NPH, Lente, Ultralente), it may be best to use only rapid-acting insulin (Humalog/Novolog) during your travel days. Otherwise, the basal insulin will peak at an inappropriate time given the time change. Plan to check your blood sugar, have a meal or snack, and take an injection of rapid-acting insulin every 3 to 4 hours. Once you reach your destination (or return home), it should be safe to resume your usual injection schedule.

Be aware that insulin outside the United States could have a different concentration than the U-100 insulin you are used to using. It is common to find U-40 insulin in some countries, which means that the insulin is only 40% as potent as U-100 insulin. If you run out of your insulin and are forced to use U-40 insulin, multiply your usual dose by 2.5. In other words, if you usually take 10 units, you will need 25 units to get the same effect. If using a pump with U-40 insulin, increase your boluses and your basals by 250% (multiply your usual doses by 2.5).

And remember, insulin is stable at room temperature for up to a month. There is not usually a need to refrigerate your insulin while traveling. However, temperatures can become dangerously high or low in luggage compartments, cars/buses, and anyplace where the outdoor climate reaches extremes. As a general rule, keep your insulin with you while traveling. If the accommodations at your destination are not adequately heated or air conditioned, bring along a thermal case for your insulin vials (MediCool, MedPort).

New Federal regulations prohibit bringing sharp objects onto airplanes. To ensure that you can travel with syringes, lancets, and other diabetes paraphernalia, bring along the original package from your insulin, including the prescription label.

Secondary Factors That Tend to Lower Blood Sugars

Aging
With advanced age comes a reduction in hormones (such as growth hormone) that counteract insulin. Even without changes in body weight or activity levels, insulin sensitivity may increase during the later years of life.

The Adjustment:
Be prepared to cut back on both basal and bolus insulin after age 60. Hypoglycemia is particularly dangerous in the elderly, due to impaired **counterregulation** (the body's hormones do little to help raise the blood sugar back toward normal in the event of a low) and the risk of falls and heart attacks. It is usually advisable to raise the target blood sugar and adjust insulin doses at the first signs of hypoglycemia.

Brain Work
The central nervous system is one of the body's major consumers of glucose. Brain cells rely almost exclusively on glucose for energy. Whenever the brain is working overtime, blood sugar levels may drop. This can occur during periods of intense concentration (studying, multitasking), adjustment to new surroundings (new job, new home), and complex social situations (hosting a party, business

networking, "working the floor"). Simply being in an environment that features lots of mental stimulation, such as a shopping center, supermarket, arcade, or casino, can make blood sugars drop.

The Adjustment:

It can be difficult to predict when brain activity is going to be high enough to induce a blood sugar drop. If you detect a *pattern* of blood sugar drops in certain situations, it makes sense to either reduce your insulin or increase your food intake in anticipation of such an event.

For example, I have a tendency to "drop while I shop." So, I try to go grocery shopping after dinner (real men shop at night), and I reduce my dinner bolus by about a third to prevent hypoglycemia. I also have a propensity for going low when I take my kids to "Chuck E. Cheese" (the loudest place on earth) to play. While I'm there, I try to graze on some carrots or other veggies (they actually have a salad bar!) to keep my blood sugar from going low.

Climate

Warm, humid temperatures have a tendency to cause blood sugar levels to drop. This is caused by accelerated absorption of insulin from below the skin as blood vessels dilate to keep the body cool. This effect is more pronounced with longer-acting insulins, including basal insulins, which can absorb more quickly and run out sooner after very hot baths or showers.

The Adjustment:

Seasonal changes may require modest (10–20%) changes in basal as well as bolus insulin doses. Short-term dosage adjustments may be needed when traveling to a climate that is warmer than what you are used to. Moving exercise from indoors to outdoors (and vice versa) may also necessitate a change in your dosage multiplier, particularly when the weather outside is very hot or cold. When taking basal insulin, try to inject into areas that will not be heated excessively by shower/bath water, or at least try to use warm rather than hot water when bathing.

High Altitude

Traveling to altitudes that are much higher than you are accustomed to can cause blood sugar levels to drop. At high altitudes, the metabolism (heart rate, respiration) increases in order to deliver enough oxygen to the body's cells. Luckily, the body usually adjusts to high altitudes within a few days, and metabolism returns to normal.

The Adjustment:

Be prepared to lower your basal insulin by 20–40% when traveling to high altitudes. This will keep your blood sugar from dropping between meals and while you sleep. Exercising at high altitudes may require a greater dosage reduction than you are used to, as the body has to work extra hard to supply enough oxygen to your muscles. After 2 or 3 days (or sooner, if you notice that your readings are coming in consistently high), return to your normal basal insulin doses.

Medications

Certain medications, including beta blockers, MAO inhibitors, nicotine patches, and antianxiety agents, may result in a temporary reduction in blood sugar levels.

The Adjustment:

Speak to the physician who prescribed the medication to determine whether the dosage warrants any up-front changes in your insulin doses. Otherwise, take a "wait and see" approach. If you notice lower-than-usual blood sugar levels after starting the medication, cut back on your insulin accordingly. If the lower readings take place at a consistent time of day, reduce your bolus insulin prior to that time. For example, if you have been going low in the afternoon since starting on a nicotine patch, reduce your lunchtime bolus. If lower readings are occurring randomly throughout the day and night, lower your basal insulin dosage in 20% increments until the problem is resolved.

Sex

Many people forget that sexual intercourse is a form of cardiovascular exercise (assuming you're doing it right!). The more prolonged and intense the lovemaking, the greater the tendency for blood sugar levels to drop.

The Adjustment:

If you can predict approximately when sex is going to take place, you could reduce your bolus at the previous meal or snack by up to 50%. If the timing (or occurrence) of sex remains a mystery, be prepared with some quick carbohydrates. Of course, subtlety is preferred. A few bite-sized chocolates might help to maintain the romantic mood better than wolfing down a giant sandwich. Of course, if you're lucky enough to have a partner who enjoys wearing edible underwear . . . you get the point.

Roller-Coaster Secondary Factors

Sometimes, the same event can cause blood sugars to rise *and* fall (or vice versa). That's why I call them roller-coaster factors. For example, consider the following:

Alcohol

Alcoholic beverages that contain carbohydrates (beer, sweet wine, frozen/mixed drinks) will raise the blood sugar in the short term. However, alcohol has a tendency to lower blood sugar levels several hours later, by suppressing the liver's normal secretion of glucose. As a result, hypoglycemia can occur several hours after drinking. The problem is made worse by the fact that intoxication often masks the symptoms of hypoglycemia. Neither the person with diabetes nor people around him/her are aware of the low blood sugar because the hypoglycemic symptoms take on the look, sound, and feel of being "drunk." Consequently, prevention of hypoglycemia is of paramount importance when drinking.

The Adjustment:

When drinking, boluses should be given to cover the carbohydrates in your beverages. However, basal insulin levels should be reduced to accommodate for the drop in blood sugar that will occur several hours later. It takes about 2 hours, on average, for each alcoholic beverage to be processed by the liver. Therefore, basal insulin should be lowered by 30–50% for 2 hours *per drink*. Four drinks? Lower the basal for 8 hours. If you take an intermediate-acting insulin at bedtime, lower the dose by 10% for each drink you had that evening, up to an 80% reduction. If you take Ultralente, Lantus, or Detemir, take the usual dose but have a snack after drinking. Ideally, the snack should be of the "low glycemic index" variety, so as to provide a steady flow of sugar into the bloodstream for several hours.

> *Alcohol tends to cause a delayed drop in blood sugar levels.*

Impaired Digestion

Gastroparesis is a form of diabetic neuropathy in which the stomach is slow to empty into the intestines, and food digests much slower than usual. Blood sugar has a tendency to rise several hours after eating rather than right after the meal.

The Adjustment:

Gastroparesis can be treated in a variety of ways. It is possible to facilitate the movement of food into the intestines with oral medications, electrical stimulation, or modifications to the diet. If these prove to be ineffective, mealtime insulin adjustments will be necessary. Switching from a rapid-acting insulin (Humalog/Novolog) to Regular insulin works for many people. Regular's delayed peak (2 to 3 hours after injection) and prolonged action (5 to 6 hours) helps to match the absorption of sugars into the bloodstream for those with impaired digestion. Another option is to delay the mealtime bolus until 30 or 60 minutes after the meal. Those who use insulin pumps can apply an "extended" or "square wave" bolus to spread the bolus delivery over a couple of hours.

Menstruation

During menstrual cycles, the body produces hormones that can raise and lower blood sugar levels. Many women find that their blood sugar levels are significantly higher a few days before the onset of their period, and lower after menses begins. Although the effects last around the clock, morning blood sugars seem to be affected the most.

The Adjustment:

Note the onset of your period in your self-monitoring records for at least three months. If you observe a pattern of consistent high or low blood sugars surrounding your menstrual cycle, adjust your insulin accordingly. Waking up high before your period? As soon as premenstrual symptoms appear, raise your overnight basal insulin by 50%. Tend to go low in the afternoon for a few days after your period begins? Try lowering your breakfast/lunch boluses by 25%.

Irregular Sleep Patterns

Difficulty sleeping can cause fluctuations in daily hormone production and may affect eating and exercise patterns. Excessive sleeping can impair the body's sensitivity to insulin, while sleep deprivation can result in heightened sensitivity to insulin.

The Adjustments:

Be prepared to increase your basal and bolus insulin if your sleep increases. Conversely, reductions in basal and bolus insulin will likely be required if you are sleeping very little.

In most cases, sleep disorders can be attributed to emotional upset or underlying illnesses. Your physician may be able to prescribe appropriate medication or refer you for counseling. Almost everyone benefits from maintaining a fairly consistent sleep/wake schedule. This usually starts with a reasonable wake-up time.

If you must deviate from your normal sleep pattern for more than a couple of days, you may need to shift the peak time of your basal insulin (if using a pump, NPH, Lente, or Ultralente insulin) so as to coincide with your body's glucose production pattern. Consider the following example:

Ben normally rises at 7 a.m., and his basal insulin normally peaks at 4 to 6 a.m. However, a change in his work schedule has him going to sleep much later and waking around noon. He is likely to need a shift in his basal insulin so that the peak occurs later in the morning rather than in the pre-dawn hours.

Bolus formula changes may also become necessary with changes in sleep patterns. The first meal of the day (i.e., breakfast) often requires a different insulin-to-carb ratio than meals consumed later in the day. If you begin sleeping until midday and lunch becomes your first meal, it would take on that "first meal" insulin-to-carb ratio.

Menopause

Natural menopause is caused by a progressive reduction in estrogen production by the ovaries. Surgical menopause occurs when the ovaries are removed, resulting in a sudden decrease in estrogen. Weight gain often accompanies menopause. Hot flashes, mood swings, and fatigue may occur as levels of estrogen ebb and flow. Because estrogen makes the body more sensitive to insulin, blood sugar control during menopause can become increasingly challenging.

Many women report more frequent and severe low blood sugars during early menopause, especially during the night. Most find that their body is more resistant to insulin and that higher doses are required in the later stages of menopause, as estrogen levels decrease permanently.

The Adjustment:

Changes in blood sugar levels during menopause are varied and highly individualized. I would hesitate to make "permanent" changes to your program until a pattern of high or low readings is established over a period of several consecutive days. Daily fluctuations in estrogen levels are common and can fool you into thinking that you need to make a change in your overall program. Try not to become overly frustrated by the seemingly senseless blood sugar variations—it is a common and natural occurrence during this phase of your life, but one that you will get through.

Pregnancy

For women with type 1 diabetes, having a baby means more than just emotional ups and downs. It also means a blood sugar roller coaster. During weeks 8 to 16 of pregnancy, insulin requirements tend to be lower than usual, followed by a gradual increase in insulin needs until the baby is delivered.

Severe hypoglycemia is three times more common during the first trimester of pregnancy than during the 4 months preceding pregnancy. This is partially due to the drive for very tight control during pregnancy, and partially due to the uptake of glucose by the growing fetus. Compounding the problem is a suppressed counter-regulatory hormone response to hypoglycemia. Traditional hypoglycemic symptoms tend to appear at lower blood sugar levels during pregnancy.

The risk of hypoglycemia is greatly increased during the first few months of pregnancy.

Following the first 16 weeks of pregnancy, the production of a number of hormones (including human placental lactogen, progesterone, prolactin, and cortisol) increases, resulting in a progressive state of insulin resistance and gradually increasing insulin requirements until the time of delivery. Immediately following delivery, insulin requirements drop precipitously; some women require little or no insulin for a day or two following delivery.

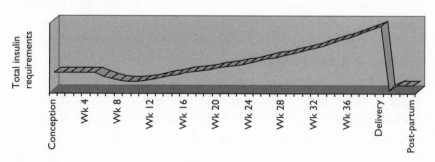

Table 8-2: Typical insulin requirements during pregnancy

The Adjustments:

Despite the drive for tighter control, insulin doses (both basal and bolus) may need to be reduced during the first 2 to 4 months following conception. Both basal and bolus insulin should be reduced in the event of repeated bouts of hypoglycemia. Conversely, both basal and bolus insulin will likely need to be increased at frequent intervals (monthly, or perhaps weekly) starting at about the 16-week point. Communicate frequently with your doctor and diabetes educator throughout your pregnancy. Adjusting quickly to meet your changing insulin requirements can make a real difference for the health of you and your baby.

Sports

In Chapter 6, the role of exercise in blood sugar regulation was dicussed in detail. Physical activity should always improve sensitivity to insulin and contribute to lower blood glucose levels. However, physical activity combined with a surge of adrenaline can result in a temporary blood sugar rise. A 2-hour soccer practice can produce much lower blood sugars than a competitive 2-hour soccer game—even when the same amount of exercise is performed.

The Adjustment:

For most athletes, "training" and "playing for fun" tend to induce a blood sugar drop. Reductions in the pre-exercise bolus are usually in order. However, competitive sports and activities that involve brief, high-intensity bursts of activity will usually induce a blood sugar rise. Increasing the pre-exercise bolus insulin will typically keep blood sugars closer to target during these types of activities.

For example, a runner may need 50% less insulin before running on her own, but 25% *more* insulin before running competitively. Don't forget: Exhaustive sporting events often produce a *delayed* blood sugar drop. A temporary reduction in basal insulin (for pump users) or a reduction in boluses for several hours following such events can help prevent delayed-onset hypoglycemia.

9

Going to Extremes

To THIS POINT, ALL attention has been focused on matching insulin to our precise needs (Thinking like a pancreas!). But let's be realistic. With so many variables and factors influencing blood sugar levels, you are going to experience your share of both high and low readings. Even the best-managed patients have readings that are out of range up to 33% of the time.

In this chapter, we will focus on what happens when the insulin we take does not meet our body's needs. When too much insulin is taken, low blood sugar (hypoglycemia) occurs. Mild forms of hypoglycemia are easily self-treated with a reduction in mealtime insulin or a modest snack. Severe forms of hypoglycemia usually require outside assistance and may lead to loss of consciousness, seizures, coma, or even death.

When too little insulin is taken, high blood sugar (hyperglycemia) occurs. Most garden-variety episodes of hyperglycemia are easily treated with correction insulin. However, a severe lack of insulin in the body can result in a life-threatening condition known as Diabetic Ketoacidosis (DKA). Since death is something we generally try to avoid, strategies for both prevention and treatment of severe hypoglycemia and DKA will be presented in this chapter.

The Science Behind Hypoglycemia

Hypoglycemia (hereafter referred to as a "low") is the main limiting factor in intensive diabetes management. Without the risk of lows, we could simply load up on insulin and never have another high reading. Or, as my wife so eloquently reminds me from time to time, "Any idiot can have a decent A1c if they're taking too much insulin and going low all the time!"

Virtually all systems of the body are affected by low blood sugar, but none quite as much as the brain. Brain cells are picky about their fuel source: They only like to burn sugar for energy. Brain and nerve cells have another special feature: They do not require insulin to get sugar inside. Instead, they have special built-in "transporters" that shuttle sugar across the cell membrane without the aid of insulin.

Low blood sugar is usually defined as a level of less than 70 mg/dl (3.9 mmol). Mild lows can cause inconvenience, embarrassment, poor physical and mental performance, impaired judgment, mood changes, weight gain, and "rebound" high blood sugars. More severe lows can induce seizures, loss of consciousness, coma, or even death. Repeated or prolonged severe hypoglycemia can result in permanent mental impairments.

Mild Lows

Soon after diabetes is diagnosed, hypoglycemia is detected quickly and easily by the central nervous system. In some cases, symptoms can occur even at blood sugars above 70 (3.9). Blood sugars in the 80s or 90s, or a rapid drop from a very high level toward a more normal level, may induce a reaction.

Upon sensing that the blood sugar is low, the brain sends a signal to the adrenal gland, which releases a surge of adrenaline. Adrenaline, in turn, stimulates the liver to secrete extra sugar into the bloodstream and temporarily inhibits the action of insulin. Adrenaline also causes a number of physical symptoms: rapid heartbeat, perspiration, shaking, hunger, and a generally anxious feeling. (You may recognize these as the same symptoms that occur when you are under intense stress.) At this point, most people are capable of thinking rationally and consuming food in order to raise their blood sugar level.

Moderate Lows

If blood sugar levels are allowed to drop into the 50s or 40s (3–2 mmol), the brain begins losing the ability to function properly. Confusion usually sets in, accompanied by dizziness and weakness. Speech may become slurred. You may exhibit unusual emotions such as irritability or despair. Vision may become blurred. You will have a difficult time thinking clearly and coordinating your movements. At this point, you may or may not be able to think rationally enough to consume food to raise your blood sugar. In many instances, a friend or family member will need to assist you.

Severe Lows

An extreme or extended blood sugar drop may cause you to pass out or experience a **seizure**. Very severe, prolonged lows can result in coma or death, although this is a rare occurrence. Severe lows will always require outside assistance and administration of glucagon (via injection) or dextrose (via an IV).

The DEVOlution of Symptoms

No, it's not a typo. And it has nothing to do with the band Devo ("Whip It," circa 1980). The symptoms of hypoglycemia do not evolve: They "devolve," or break down, over time. The brain has a propensity for becoming more efficient at extracting glucose from the bloodstream after going years with off-and-on low blood sugars. In other words, mild low blood sugars will cease to be detected by the brain; little or no adrenaline response is produced, and physical symptoms (shaking, sweating, etc.) fail to take place. Thus, there may be no warning of low blood sugar in its early stages. The first symptoms are those of a moderate low blood sugar (confusion, etc.), and these may not occur until the blood sugar is already at a dangerously low level (40s or less).

The name given to this phenomenon is **"hypoglycemia unawareness."** It affects most people who have had diabetes for several years or more, and tends to become worse over time. The more lows you get, the less likely you are to get any warning signs the next time. Quite a paradox!

> *Meticulous prevention of low blood sugars for several weeks may help restore early warning signs of low blood sugar.*

Research has shown that the early symptoms of low blood sugar can be restored (at least to some extent) by avoiding lows over an extended period of time. People with severe cases of hypoglycemia unawareness have been able to reestablish their early warning symptoms by going several weeks without any readings below 80 (4.4). While this process may require a temporary increase in the HbA1c level, it is well worth it to help prevent severe hypoglycemia.

Treatment of Lows

Diabetes is a tricky disease. Low blood sugars sometimes feel like highs, and highs sometimes feel like lows. If you suspect that your blood sugar is low, take a few seconds to confirm it by checking your blood sugar. I can't tell you how many times I thought I was low, only to test and get a reading in the 200s (12–17). High blood sugars can cause symptoms similar to those caused by lows (tiredness, hunger, a "jittery" feeling). Getting an exact reading will also help to determine how much carb you need to treat the low.

With pre-meal blood sugars that are below your target but above 70 mg/dl (3.9 mmol), it is usually best to reduce your meal bolus using your correction formula. For readings below 70, it is best to treat the low immediately, wait 10 to 15 minutes for the blood sugar to come up, and then have your meal (giving the usual dose for your meal).

There is no one-size-fits-all treatment for hypoglycemia. Proper treatment depends on a number of factors, including the following:

1. Body Size: The bigger you are, the more carbs it will take to raise your blood sugar. If you weigh less than 60 pounds (28 kg), each gram of carbohydrate should raise your blood sugar about 6–8 mg/dl (0.33–0.44 mmol); if you weigh 60 to 100 pounds (29–47 kg), each gram should raise it about 5 mg/dl (0.28); at 101 to 160 pounds (48–76 kg), the rise is about 4 points (0.22); 161 to 220 pounds (77–105 kg): about 3 pts (0.17); over 220 pounds (105 kg): 2 pts (0.11).

2. Blood Sugar Level: The lower your blood sugar, the more carbs you will need to get back up to normal. Table 9-1, below, provides a good starting point. The goal on this chart is to raise the blood sugar to about 120 mg/dl (6.7 mmol). If your specific blood sugar target is more or less than 120, you will need more or fewer carbs than the amount listed.

   Carbs needed to raise blood sugar to approximately 120 mg/dl (6.7 mmol):

Blood Sugar	60s (3.3–3.9)	50s (2.8–3.2)	40s (2.2–2.7)	30s (1.7–2.1)	20s (1.1–1.6)
Weight: <60 lbs (28 kg)	9g	11g	13g	15g	17g
60–100 lbs (29–47 kg)	11g	13g	15g	17g	19g
101–160 lbs (48–76 kg)	14g	16g	19g	21g	24g
161–220 lbs (77–105 kg)	18g	22g	25g	28g	32g
>220 (>105 kg)	28g	33g	38g	43g	48g

Table 9-1: Proper treatment for low blood sugar (based on body weight)

The following formula can be used to determine your precise carb needs:

Grams of carb needed to treat a low =
$$\text{(Target BG} - \text{Actual BG)} \, / \, \text{Rise per gram of carb}$$

For example, if your target is 100, your blood sugar is 62, and each gram of carb raises you 3 points, you will need $(100 - 62) / 3$, or 13 g carb.

3. Anticipated Blood Sugar Change: If you expect your blood sugar to continue dropping over the next hour, you will need more carbs than the amounts noted above. For example, if your mealtime insulin is only 1 or 2 hours old, or if you have just finished an exercise session, you should consume more carbs than the amount listed on the chart. Conversely, if you expect your blood sugar to rise soon (after a high-fat meal, for example), you may need less carbs than the amounts listed.

Remember, all carbs are not created equally. Some will raise your blood sugar very quickly, while others will take their sweet time (excuse the play on words). When your blood sugar is low, choose a food that will raise you as quickly as possible. Refer to the glycemic index and select foods with a score of at least 70. Examples of high-glycemic index foods that are portable and measurable include:

- Glucose tablets (102)

- Dry cereal (70–90)

- Pretzels (81)

- Jelly beans (80)

- Gatorade (78)

- Vanilla wafers (77)

- Graham crackers (74)

- Plain bread/crackers (70–75)

- LifeSavers (70)

Foods with a lower glycemic index, such as fruit, juice, milk, ice cream, and (hate to say it) chocolate, are not the best choices for treating lows. They will take significantly longer to raise your blood sugar level. Many people overtreat their lows by continuing to eat until the symptoms disappear. It usually takes 10 to 15 minutes for *high* glycemic index foods to raise the blood sugar, and 20 to 60 minutes for *low* glycemic foods. Be patient! If you suspect that your blood sugar has not come up enough, test it to find out. If your blood sugar is still below 70 (3.9) 15 minutes after treatment, go ahead and eat a little bit more.

> *Resist the temptation to overtreat your lows. If you do overtreat, take some fast-acting insulin to cover the excess carbs.*

If you happen to go overboard on the treatment of your low (as we all do on occasion), cover the excess carbs with insulin. For example, if you normally take 1 unit for every 10 grams of carb and you overtreat your low by 40 grams, give yourself 4 units of insulin once your blood sugar has risen back to normal. Otherwise, your blood sugar will rise well above your target.

Treating Severe Lows

Severe hypoglycemia (when a person is unwilling or unable to consciously swallow food) must be treated differently than mild and moderate lows. It is dangerous to put any kind of food into the mouth of someone having a severe low. They could choke on the food and suffocate, or they could instinctively bite down and take the fingers off the person trying to feed them.

There are two things, and only two things, you should do to treat someone having a severe low blood sugar: Call for emergency help, and administer an injection of glucagon.

Glucagon is a hormone (like insulin) that raises blood sugar by stimulating the liver to release its stored-up sugar into the bloodstream. It will usually work in 10 to 20 minutes. Glucagon is a prescription item that comes in a kit containing a large fluid-filled syringe, a small vial with the glucagon hormone in powder form, and instructions written in a seemingly foreign language. The kits have an expiration date (they are usually good for about 2 years), so check them periodically to make sure yours is fresh. If possible, save your expired kits and use them for practice (on a foam ball, not your spouse!).

The procedure for administering glucagon, in PLAIN ENG-LISH, is as follows:

1. Call 911. Have paramedics on the way in case the glucagon injection fails to work.

2. Pull the cap off the syringe and flip the cap off the vial.

3. Inject all of the fluid into the vial.

4. Remove the syringe from the vial. Keep pressure on the plunger to make sure air does not escape from the vial.

5. Shake the vial until the fluid is evenly mixed (no clumps) and mostly clear.

6. With the vial held upside down, reinsert the *tip* of the needle into the vial. (Do NOT put the whole needle in; you will draw in air accidentally!)

7. Draw the fluid into the syringe. For very small children (under age 6), draw in ⅓ cc; for children 6 to 12, draw in ½ cc; over age 12, draw in 1 cc.

8. Insert the needle straight (not at an angle) into a muscle such as the thigh, buttocks, or back of the arm. Inject the full contents of the syringe.

9. Remove the syringe and apply a tissue to suppress any bleeding.

10. Turn the victim onto his or her side to prevent choking (in case vomiting occurs).

The victim should regain consciousness in 10 to 20 minutes. If he or she does do not, wait for paramedics to arrive. Contact your health care team to troubleshoot and work on a plan for preventing the severe low from happening again.

Note: Everyone who takes insulin is at risk for severe hypoglycemia. It is important to wear medical identification (Medic Alert) at all times. The Medic Alert Foundation provides more than just medical I.D. jewelry: It maintains a database of medical information that paramedics will have instant access to when they call in. Bracelets and necklaces are recommended because these are the first things paramedics will look for when they arrive at the scene.

Prevention of Lows

Minimizing the incidence of low blood sugar can go a long way in terms of protecting your personal safety and keeping blood sugar levels from bouncing around too much as a result of rebounds. As mentioned earlier, it is also the best way to ensure that you will experience symptoms when your blood sugar is dropping and thus be able to treat the low before it becomes severe.

It is usually acceptable to experience two or three mild low blood sugars per week. If they are occurring more often, or if they are of a severe nature, try applying these strategies:

Match Insulin to Needs

The first step in preventing lows is the same as the first step in achieving tight control—mimic the action of a healthy pancreas as closely as possible. Daytime doses of NPH, Lente, or Ultralente do not match the basal/bolus insulin secretion of the pancreas as well as programs that utilize basal insulin. These types of insulin can peak at inconsistent and inappropriate times, increasing the odds of low blood sugar. Nighttime doses can also peak unpredictably, causing nocturnal hypoglycemia. Switching to a basal insulin

(Lantus, Detemir, or an insulin pump) will greatly reduce your risk for hypoglycemia.

Use Rapid-Acting Insulin

Rapid-acting insulin analogs (Humalog, Novolog) tend to produce fewer low blood sugars than Regular insulin. Their rapid onset, consistent peak, and short duration of action match up well to the absorption of carbohydrates in most meals. Regular insulin peaks later and lasts significantly longer. It has a tendency to make blood sugars drop 3 to 6 hours after eating—long after the food has been digested and absorbed.

Dose Properly

Accidental overdosing of insulin is a common cause of hypo-glycemia. If you are on relatively low doses (less than 5 units per injection), look for syringes (Becton-Dickinson) or pens (Novo Nordisk, Becton Dickinson) that offer half-unit markings, so that you can dose more precisely. If you have difficulty seeing your syringes, use an insulin pen, MagniGuide (Becton-Dickinson), or Count-A-Dose (Palco Labs). If necessary, have someone else draw up your syringes. And PAY ATTENTION TO YOUR MATH! A single incorrect calculation can send your blood sugar spiraling downward. If you accidentally take too much insulin, drink enough carbs to offset the extra dose, and check your blood sugar hourly until the insulin wears off.

Give Your Insulin Time to Work

As I mentioned in Chapter 7, boluses of rapid-acting insulin do not stop working after just an hour or 2. They typically take 3 or 4 hours to finish working. When figuring the amount of correction insulin required to reduce a high blood sugar, it is important to take the unused portion of your previous boluses into account.

Time Your Boluses Properly

Foods that have a low glycemic index value tend to take a while to raise the blood sugar level. Very large meals that contain a great deal of protein or fat can also take a while to raise the blood sugar. Giving a bolus before or during these types of meals can cause low blood sugar soon after eating. Instead, plan to give your boluses *after* eating or, if using an insulin pump, program the bolus to be delivered over an extended period of time.

Set Appropriate Targets

The lower your target blood sugar, the greater your chances for going low. Target blood sugars of 80 or 90 (4.4–5.0) leave little margin for error. Even the slightest bit of extra exercise or a minor overestimate of carbohydrates will probably result in a low. A target of 100 (5.6) or more allows a bit more "breathing room."

Time Meals and Snacks Appropriately

When using any type of intermediate- or long-acting insulin, it is imperative that you consume your meals and snacks so as to coincide with the peak action time of the insulin. A delay of as little as half an hour can cause a sharp drop in blood sugar. If you anticipate a delay of 15 minutes or more, consume part of your usual meal or snack, in the form of a carbohydrate-containing beverage.

Discount Fiber Grams

Don't forget: Fiber is included in the total carbohydrate listing on food labels, but it does not raise blood sugar levels. Any time you are consuming a food item that contains more than 2 or 3 grams of fiber, subtract it from the total carbohydrate before calculating your meal bolus.

Adjust for Exercise and Daily Activity

Physical activity of almost any kind (from running laps to running a vacuum) will accelerate the uptake of glucose by muscle cells. In those without diabetes, insulin secretion comes to a grinding halt and production of counter-regulatory hormones increases at the onset of exercise. This helps to maintain blood sugars within normal limits. For those who take insulin, adjustments must be made to prevent low blood sugars during and after exercise. For activity performed after a meal, a reduction in the meal bolus is usually in order. Activity before or between meals will require an extra snack. Prolonged or very strenuous activity may require reductions in basal and bolus insulin, along with periodic snacks before, during, and after to prevent a delayed blood sugar drop.

Adjust for Alcohol

In Chapter 8, I discussed how alcohol can cause a delayed drop in blood sugar by suppressing the liver's secretion of glucose. After drinking, be sure to either lower your basal insulin level for several hours, or consume extra snacks to compensate.

Test, Test, Test

Very few of us are good at guessing our blood sugar levels with much precision, especially when the readings are not particularly high or low. Frequent blood glucose testing will allow you to catch below-target readings before they turn into hypoglycemia. For instance, a bedtime reading of 82 (4.6) may seem innocuous, but even a slight drop during the night would result in a low blood sugar. *Knowing* that the reading is 82 allows you the opportunity to have a small snack, thus reducing the likelihood of a nighttime low.

Try a Continuous Monitor

Presently, two devices allow us to collect a wealth of blood sugar data that can be used in the prevention of low blood sugars. The GlucoWatch Biographer (Cygnus) alerts the user of a pending low by alarming whenever it detects a reading that is below a threshold set by the user. Its data recall can also indicate patterns and trends during the night. Likewise, the Continuous Glucose Monitoring System (Medtronic/MiniMed) records readings every 5 minutes for a 72-hour period for subsequent analysis. The data and charts produced by the CGMS can indicate undetected lows during the night or between meals, so that appropriate changes to insulin doses can be made.

The Other Extreme: Ketoacidosis

DKA (Diabetic Ketoacidosis) is a condition in which the blood becomes highly acidic as a result of dehydration and excessive ketone (acid) production. When bodily fluids become acidic, certain systems stop functioning properly. It is a serious condition that will make you violently ill and can kill you. The primary cause of DKA is a lack of working insulin in the body. Let me explain.

Normal Fuel Metabolism

Most of the body's cells burn primarily sugar (glucose) for energy. Many cells also burn fat, but in much smaller amounts. Glucose happens to be a very "clean" form of energy. It's like natural gas— there are virtually no pollutants produced when you burn it up. Fat, on the other hand, is a "dirty" source of energy. When fat is burned, there are waste products produced. These waste products are called "ketones." Ketones are acid molecules that can pollute the bloodstream if produced in large quantities. Luckily, we don't tend to burn huge amounts of fat at one time, and the ketones that are produced can be broken down during the process of glucose metabolism. Glucose and ketones can "jump into the fire" together.

As you can tell, it is important to have an ample supply of glucose in the body's cells. That requires two things: sugar (glucose) in the bloodstream, and *insulin* to shuttle the sugar into the cells (see Figure 9-1).

Abnormal Fuel Metabolism

What would happen if you had no insulin? I'm not talking about a minor under-dosage; I'm talking about having virtually no insulin whatsoever. A number of things would start to go wrong. Without insulin, glucose cannot get into the body's cells. As a result, the cells begin burning large amounts of fat for energy. This, of course, leads to the production of large amounts of ketones. Although some of the ketones eventually spill over into the urine, the body is unable to eliminate sufficient amounts to restore a healthy pH balance in the bloodstream (see Figure 9-2, page 189).

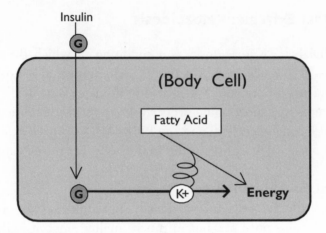

G=Glucose; K+=Ketone

Figure 9-1: Cellular metabolism in the presence of insulin

The problem is further complicated by dehydration. Without sufficient insulin to inhibit the liver's secretion of sugar, large amounts of glucose are released into the bloodstream. Because high blood sugar causes excessive urination, dehydration ensues. Without glucose metabolism to help break down the ketones, and without ample fluids to help neutralize the ketones, the bloodstream and tissues of the body become very acidic (see Figure 9-3, page 190). This is a state of ketoacidosis.

Causes and Prevention of Ketoacidosis

What can cause a sudden lack of insulin in the body? There are a number of potential culprits.

Illness, Infection, and Dehydration

Illness, infection, and dehydration can cause the production of large quantities of stress hormones, which counteract insulin. In other words, during an illness, you could have insulin in your body, but it is rendered almost useless because stress hormones are blocking its action.

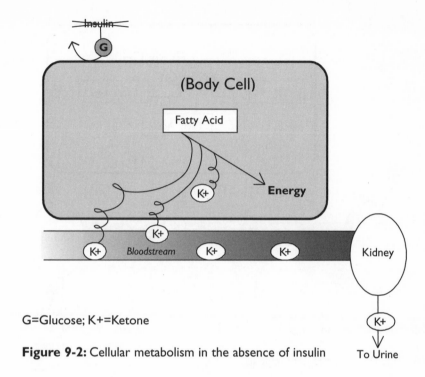

G=Glucose; K+=Ketone

Figure 9-2: Cellular metabolism in the absence of insulin

Prevention:

The sick-day strategies presented in Chapter 8 are worth repeating. During an illness, insulin requirements are usually increased—even if you are not eating as much as usual. Keep taking your basal insulin regardless of your food intake. If your blood sugars are running high or if ketones are present in your urine, you may need to increase your dose of basal insulin by as much as 200%.

Lack of Carbohydrates

Ketone production can also be induced by a lack of carbohydrates in the diet. During periods of starvation, prolonged fasting, or restricted carbohydrate intake, the body's cells must resort to burning alternative sources of fuel: namely fat and protein. With increased fat metabolism and limited carbohydrate metabolism, ketone production may exceed the body's ability to eliminate them.

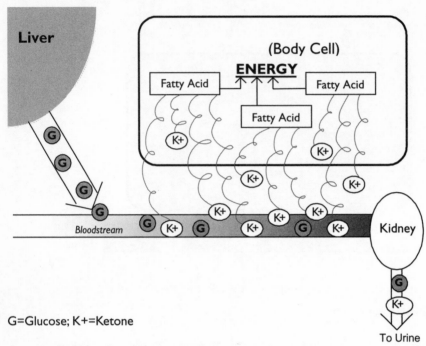

G=Glucose; K+=Ketone

Figure 9-3: The onset of ketoacidosis

Prevention:

Ketone production is unhealthy for anyone, particularly those with diabetes. Maintaining at least a modest level of carbohydrate intake throughout the day should prevent ketosis. If you must fast for short periods of time, talk with your doctor to ensure that it will not interfere with any other health conditions or medications that you may be taking.

Fasting can usually be accomplished safely by taking only basal insulin, with rapid-acting insulin as touch-ups for high blood sugars. If you take an intermediate-acting insulin in the morning, take half of your usual dose. Be sure to check your blood sugar level regularly during a fast. If your blood sugar drops below 70 (3.9), you must snack to bring it back up.

Spoiled Insulin

Using spoiled insulin can lead to high blood sugar and ketone production. Insulin that has been exposed to extreme cold or heat can "denature," or break down so that the insulin molecules no longer work. Using the same vial or cartridge of insulin over many months, or using it past its expiration date can also result in spoilage.

Prevention:

Insulin vials and cartridges should not be used after their expiration date. Once you begin using a vial or cartridge, it should be discarded after 1 month. Keep your unopened insulin stored in the refrigerator, in an area that is not likely to freeze (the butter compartment works great for me). Before using a new vial or cartridge, look for "clumps," crystals on the glass, or discoloration. If you suspect that the insulin has gone bad, it probably has. When ordering insulin by mail, ask that it be shipped in a temperature-controlled container. Keep your insulin in your carry-on when you travel, as luggage may be exposed to extreme cold temperatures.

Poor Absorption

Poor absorption at the injection site can also cause an insulin deficiency. Remember, once insulin is injected or infused under the skin, it must absorb into the bloodstream in order to take effect. If the insulin "pockets" under the skin, it may never actually work. In some cases, the insulin may absorb much later than expected, resulting in a high blood sugar followed by an unanticipated low.

Prevention:

Just as you rotate your tires to prevent uneven tread wear, you must rotate your injection and infusion (pump) sites to prevent uneven insulin absorption. Injecting the same spots repeatedly can cause **lipodystrophy**—a breakdown or inflammation of the fat tissue below the skin. When this happens, the skin can either dimple or become unusually hard and insensitive. One of my patients calls these "happy spots" because they don't hurt at all when giving a shot or inserting an infusion set. The problem with happy spots is that they tend to have reduced blood flow, and insulin does not absorb properly—if at all. Avoid giving insulin into these areas. Spreading your injection and infusion sites over a large area of skin should help prevent the development of lipodystrophy. And with the exception of NPH, Lente, and Ultralente, insulin may (and should) be given in a variety of body parts, including the thighs, abdomen, buttocks, and backs of the arms.

Missed Injections

Missed or omitted injections are another potential cause of an insulin deficiency. Missing an occasional meal bolus will not typically cause the body to become totally devoid of insulin, but missed basal insulin injections or repeated missed boluses can have serious consequences.

Prevention:

Plan to take your basal insulin at about the same time each day. If possible, combine it with another activity, such as brushing your teeth, taking oral medication, or eating a certain meal. Getting into a routine is the best way to ensure that critical basal insulin injections will not be missed. Users of the latest insulin pumps can avoid missing boluses by programming "missed bolus reminders" at key times of day. Those who take injections might have an easier time remembering to bolus if blood sugars are taken at each meal/snack time and if written records are being kept.

Gaps in Coverage

An insulin program that has *"gaps" in insulin coverage* or is *grossly deficient* in the total amount of insulin could also induce ketone production and ketoacidosis.

Prevention:

It is reasonable to question your doctor's insulin dosage recommendations if (1) there is no basal insulin component to your program, or (2) the total amount of insulin for the day is less than 0.5 units per kilogram of your body weight (if you have type 1 diabetes) or less than 0.25 units per kilogram of your body weight (if you have type 2 diabetes).

Insulin Pump Malfunction

Insulin pump therapy opens the door to ketoacidosis in the event of a problem with insulin delivery, absorption, or action. With no intermediate- or long-acting insulin in the body, pumpers rely on the pump's delivery of basal insulin in the form of tiny pulses of rapid-acting insulin. Any interruption in insulin delivery can result in a sharp rise in blood sugar and ketone production starting as soon as 3 hours after the last bit of insulin was infused. This can be caused by any of the following:

- tubing or infusion set clogs;

- leaks where the cartridge connects to the tubing;

- air pockets in the tubing;

- dislodgement of the **canula**/infusion set tube from the skin;

- improper or insufficient priming;

- extended pump suspension; or

- extended disconnection or forgetting to reconnect.

The best way for pump users to prevent ketoacidosis is to test for ketones with any unusually high readings. If ketones are present, inject insulin with a syringe, drink plenty of water, and change the pump's cartridge and infusion set.

Prevention:

The first and most important step in preventing ketoacidosis when using an insulin pump is early detection of a problem. This is accomplished by checking for ketones with any unusually high blood sugar levels. The absence of ketones indicates that the high reading is probably due to insufficient insulin coverage for food eaten recently. The presence of ketones indicates either an illness/infection or, more likely, a problem with the pump's insulin delivery.

Three steps should reverse the problem if ketones are present:

I. Give an injection of insulin using a syringe (using your normal correction formula to determine the dose).

2. Drink as much water as possible.

3. Change your pump's cartridge, tubing, and infusion set, using a *fresh vial of insulin*.

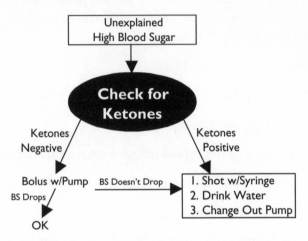

Figure 9-4: Troubleshooting with the pump

Failure to correct the problem could result in ketoacidosis in just a few hours.

To prevent insulin delivery problems with your pump, watch for the following:

• Limit your disconnection and "suspension" periods to no more than an hour at a time. If you must disconnect for more than an hour, reconnect hourly and bolus an amount equal to the basal insulin that you missed in the previous hour.

• Check your infusion site and tubing at least once daily. If the infusion set tape is peeling loose or if you spot any blood in the canula, replace the infusion set immediately.

• Check for air pockets in the tubing each day; if you spot any, disconnect and prime until the air has been purged completely out.

- If you smell insulin or detect moisture around any of the joints where the tubing connects to the pump or infusion set, replace them immediately.

- If your pump alerts you of a tubing/infusion set clog ("no delivery," "occlusion," "blockage detected"), replace your cartridge, tubing, and infusion set immediately. Do not just "jiggle" your infusion set and attempt to bolus again. Pumps only detect clogs after a significant amount of pressure has built up. Jiggling may temporarily help insulin flow through, but the problem is likely to reoccur.

- Change your cartridge as soon as possible after you receive your "low cartridge" warning. This minimizes the risk that your cartridge will run out completely.

Symptoms and Treatment of DKA

Everyone with diabetes who uses insulin should have a way to test for ketones. Ketone testing can be done by way of a urine dipstick (ketostix or ketodiastix) or a fingerstick blood sample (Precision Xtra meter from Abbott Labs).
"Positive" ketones are indicated by either of the following:

- Urine testing that indicates small or more ketones ($\geq$15 mg/dl)

- Blood testing that indicates the presence of ß-Hydroxybutyrate ($\geq$0.6 mmol / l)

Be sure to have fresh ketone testing supplies on hand at all times—including when you travel. Ketostix in vials are only good for 6 months after the vial has been opened. Individually foil-wrapped ketostix (Bayer) are good until their expiration date. Ketone test strips for the Precision Xtra are also foil-wrapped, but once again, they are only good until the expiration date stamped on the package.

The presence of ketones in the blood is referred to as "ketosis"; ketones in the urine is "ketonuria." Ketosis/ketonuria is usually (but not always) accompanied by elevated blood sugar, thirst, and excessive urination. This is a precursor to the more severe state of DKA. Symptoms of DKA are more pronounced. With DKA, you are likely to be nauseous or vomiting. Your breathing may be very deep, and you could have a fruity odor on your breath as your lungs try to eliminate ketones as you exhale. You will likely be dehydrated due to all the urination (as a result of the very high blood sugars). This will give you dry skin, intense thirst, and a dry mouth. Your vision may also be blurry. Headache and muscle aches are common.

> *Call your doctor immediately if you have symptoms of DKA.*

Call your doctor immediately if you have ketones in your blood or urine, or are experiencing these types of symptoms. Although fluids and insulin are the preferred form of treatment, DKA is not something that you can treat on your own. The severe dehydration that accompanies DKA usually keeps insulin from absorbing properly from below the skin. Nausea/vomiting may also limit the amount of fluid you can consume. Treatment of DKA almost always requires a visit to an emergency room for intravenous administration of insulin, water, and electrolytes. The acidity of your blood will have to be monitored very carefully at the hospital to prevent the onset of coma or sudden death. Your length of your hospital stay will vary depending on the severity of the DKA, but expect to be there for at least a day or two.

There are a few things that you can do on your own prior to hospitalization. Try to eat light, easy-to-digest carbohydrates and drink at least 8 ounces of liquid per hour. Diluted orange juice is a good choice, because it replaces fluids as well as potassium that was lost with excess urination. Check your blood sugar and ketones every couple of hours, and report the information to your doctor.

Remember: They don't call it "insulin-*dependent*" diabetes for nothing. We depend on insulin to stay alive. DKA causes more than 80% of hospital admissions for people with insulin-dependent diabetes. Practice the preventive measures described above, and stay in close contact with your health care team at the first signs of trouble.

10

Resources

Giving Support, Getting Support

FEELING THE UPS AND downs of blood sugar swings. Handling the incessant responsibilities of managing a chronic disease. Trying to make sense out of a highly "imperfect" science. And facing the grim reality that, despite all your best efforts, serious health problems may be in your future.

Living with diabetes can be a frightening and frustrating experience. At times, it can also seem very lonely.

If you have ever felt the need to reach out to someone who understands how you feel (someone who has *been there*), support networks may be just the answer. Even if you don't feel the need to receive support yourself, the act of giving support to others is worth its weight in gold. Nothing will make you feel better and enrich your life more than helping others.

Opportunities for giving and getting support are widespread. At my practice alone, we coordinate four diabetes support groups: one for insulin pump wearers, one for parents of children with diabetes, one for those trying to lose weight, and one focusing on research updates. Yet, the demand is growing for more extensive and specialized groups.

People who never pictured themselves as the "support group" type keep coming back because of how much they learn and how they come away feeling like part of a strong, united group. There are bound to be similar groups in your area: Check in your phone book or with your local hospital. Call one of the major diabetes organizations (see the listings below) to inquire about local chapters and programs.

If nothing exists near you, or if what exists fails to meet your needs, consider starting a group of your own. Post some fliers at doctors' offices, and let your local ADA and JDRF chapters know so that they can include it in their newsletters. Have the meeting at your home or at a centrally located restaurant. You could also ask a social worker at a nearby hospital if there is a room you can use. Each meeting should include plenty of networking/socializing time, but also try to have at least one pertinent topic to address. Have a sign-in sheet so that you can compile a mail (and e-mail) list for future meetings. Do not go overboard in terms of expenses for the meetings. Remember: It is the people in attendance that are the highlight. Light snacks and beverages are more than enough. As the group grows, you might consider bringing in guest speakers from various hospitals or pharmaceutical companies, and asking them to sponsor the meeting by covering your out-of-pocket costs.

For example, we hold our weight-loss support group meetings at our office once a month. The meeting is led by our registered dietitian, who opens up the meeting to any topics that the attendees want to discuss. Often, the latest "diet craze" is a hot topic, but each meeting also has a pre-advertised seasonal topic such as "handling holiday buffets," "spring into exercise," or "hints for healthy barbecuing." Once, she brought in a guest speaker specializing in eating disorders to talk about binge eating. Bottled water and diet sodas are provided for the attendees. A mailing is sent out every 3 months to all past attendees as well as anyone who has expressed interest in the meetings, detailing the topics for the next 3 months. A diabetes mail-order pharmacy helps to cover our costs, so we put out their literature at all of the meetings.

If face-to-face groups are not feasible because of space, distance, or confidentiality issues, consider participating in (or starting) a chat room on the Internet. Although information derived from chat rooms may not always be accurate, you can still gain an emotional lift from conversing with other people facing similar challenges.

Diabetes support groups range from very general to highly specific. Some are intended for anyone and everyone with a link to diabetes, while others are geared toward those with specific interests or complications.

Below is a listing of companies and organizations that offer *support, programs,* and *information* for people with diabetes.

General Organizations

American Association of Diabetes Educators (AADE)
800–338–3633
www.aadenet.org

American Diabetes Association (ADA)
800–232–3472
www.diabetes.org

American Dietetic Association (also ADA)
800–877–1600
www.eatright.org

Diabetes Camping Association (DCA)
256–883–2556
www.diabetescamps.org

Diabetes Exercise and Sports Association (DESA)
800–898–4322
www.diabetes-exercise.org

International Association for Medical Assistance to Travelers (IAMAT)
716–754–4883
www.iamat.org

The Jewish Diabetes Association (JDA)
718–787–4532
www.jewishdiabetes.org

Juvenile Diabetes Research Foundation International
(JDRFI)
800–533–CURE
www.jdrf.org

Complication-Specific Support

American Association of Kidney Patients
800–749–2257
www.aakp.org

American Celiac Society
973–325–8837
amerceliacsoc@netscape.net

American Chronic Pain Association
800–533–3231
www.theacpa.org

American Foundation for the Blind
800–232–5463
www.afb.org

American Heart Association
800–242–8721
www.amhrt.org

Amputee Coalition of America
888–267–5669
www.amputee-coalition.org

Celiac Sprue Association/USA
402–558–0600
www.csaceliacs.org

Gluten Intolerance Group of North America
206–246–6652
www.gluten.net

National Federation of the Blind Materials Resource Center
410–659–9314
www.nfb.org

National Kidney Foundation
800–622–9010
www.kidney.org

National Library Service for the Blind and Physically
Handicapped
800–424–8567
www.lcweb.loc.gov/nls

National Oral Health Information Clearinghouse
301–402–7364
www.nidr.nih.gov

Neuropathy Association
800–247–6968
www.neuropathy.org

Government Entities
National Diabetes Education Program
800–GET–LEVEL
www.niddk.nih.gov/health/diabetes/ndep/ndep.htm

National Diabetes Information Clearinghouse
800–860–8747
www.niddk.nih.gov

National Institute of Diabetes and Digestive and Kidney
Diseases
301–496–3583
www.niddk.nih.gov

National Institute of Health
301–496–4261
www.nih.gov

Journals

Countdown (the Juvenile Diabetes Research Foundation)
800–533–2873
www.jdrf.org

Diabetes Forecast (the American Diabetes Association)
800–806–7801
www.diabetes.org/diabetesforecast/

Diabetes Interview (King's Publishing)
800–488–8468
www.diabetesinterview.com

Diabetes Positive! (Positive Health Publications)
941–795–7594

Diabetes Self-Management (Rapaport Publishing)
800–234–0923
www.diabetesselfmanagement.com

Diabetes Wellness News
(Diabetes Research & Wellness Foundation)
877–633–3976
www.diabeteswellness.net

Diabetic Cooking (Publications International)
800–777–5582
www.fbnr.com

Voice of the Diabetic (the Diabetes Action Network of the National Federation of the Blind)
410–659–9314
www.nfb.org/voice.htm

Carb Counting/Nutrition Books

(many are available at Gary Scheiner's Web site: www.integrateddiabetes.com)

The Diabetes Carbohydrate and Fat Gram Guide
(the American Diabetes Association)
800–232–6733
www.store.diabetes.org

The Doctor's Pocket Calorie, Fat & Carbohydrate Counter
(Family Health Publications)
949–642–8500
www.calorieking.com

Nutrition in the Fast Lane (Franklin Publishing)
800–634–1993
www.fastfoodfacts.com

Fast Food Facts (International Diabetes Center)
888–637–2675
www.idcpublishing.com

Web Sites

Celiac's Disease (information and chat rooms)
www.celiac.com

Children With Diabetes (for kids and parents)
www.childrenwithdiabetes.com

Gary Scheiner's Diabetes Web Site:
www.integrateddiabetes.com

Insulin Pumpers (for pump users and those interested in pump therapy)
www.insulin-pumpers.org

Kids with Diabetes:
www.kidswithdiabetes.org

Rick Mendosa's Web Site (various resources and information):
www.medosa.com/diabetes.htm

Kids R Pumping
www.member.aol.com/camelsRFun/index.html

Diabetes Mall (various diabetes products and resources)
www.diabetesnet.com

Insulin Free World (info on the latest research and treatment)
www.diabetesportal.com

Diabetes Station (ongoing programs/chats on current diabetes topics)
www.diabetesstation.com

Sources of Supplies

Want more details on a product you are currently using? Curious about that new meter you saw in an advertisement? Looking to order something for the first time? Below is a listing of many prominent manufacturers and suppliers of diabetes-related products:

Insulin Pump Companies

Animas Corporation (IR-1000 and IR-1200 insulin pumps)
877–937–7867
www.animascorp.com

Dana Diabecare USA (DANA insulin pump)
866–342–2322
www.theinsulinpump.com

Disetronic Medical Systems, Inc. (H-Tron and D-Tron insulin pumps)
800–280–7801
www.disetronic-usa.com

MiniMed, Inc. (Paradigm insulin pump and the Continuous Glucose Monitoring System)
800–646–4633
www.minimed.com

Nipro Diabetes Systems (Amigo insulin pump)
888–651–PUMP
www.glucopro.com

Pump Wear Inc. (insulin pump accessories)
866–470–PUMP
www.pumpwearinc.com

Smith/Deltec, Inc. (Cozmo insulin pump)
800–426–2448
www.delteccozmo.com

Unique Pump Accessories (insulin pump accessories)
800–831–8929
www.uniaccs.com

Blood Glucose Monitoring

Abbott Labs (Medisense blood glucose meters)
800–527–3339
www.medisense.com

Bayer Health Care
(ketostix and Ascensia blood glucose meters)
800–348–8100
www.bayercarediabetes.com

Cygnus, Inc. (GlucoWatch Biographer)
866–459–2824
www.cygn.com

LifeScan, Inc. (One Touch blood glucose meters)
800–227–8862
www.lifescan.com

Roche Diagnostics (Accu-chek blood glucose meters)
800–858–8072
www.roche.com

TheraSense (freestyle blood glucose meters)
888–522–5226
www.therasense.com

Insulin Manufacturers

Aventis Pharmeceuticals (Lantus insulin)
800–981–2491
www.aventis.com

Eli Lilly and Company (insulin, insulin pens, and glucagon)
800–545–5979
www.lillydiabetes.com

Novo Nordisk Pharmaceuticals (insulin and insulin pens)
800–727–6500
www.novonordisk-us.com

Miscellaneous

Activa Brand Products
(AdvantaJet needle-free insulin infuser)
800–991–4464
www.advantajet.com

Antares Pharma, Inc. (MediJect needle-free insulin infuser)
800–328–3074
www.antarespharma.com

Becton Dickinson / BD (syringes, lancets, glucose tablets, and
self-care accessories)
888–BD–CARES
www.bddiabetes.com

FlexSite Diagnostics (home A1c and microalbumin
test kits)
877–212–8378
www.flexsite.com

Lighthouse Inc (low-vision products)
800–453–4923
www.goldviolin.com

LS&S Group (products for the visually and hearing impaired)
800–468–4789
www.lssproducts.com

Medic Alert Foundation (medical identification jewelry and a
database of health information on all members)
800–432–5378
www.medicalert.org

Medicool, Inc. (insulin injection aids; storage/travel cases for
insulin, medication, and supplies)
800–433–2469
www.medicool.com

MEDport
(storage/travel cases for insulin, medication, and supplies)
800–858–8840
www.medportinc.com

Metrika, Inc (home A1c test kit)
877–METRIKA
www.metrika.com

Palco Labs
(insulin injection aids and miscellaneous accessories)
800–346–4488
www.palcolabs.com

Glossary

Adrenaline A collection of hormones secreted by the adrenal gland in response to physical or emotional stress.

Analog Insulin Human insulin whose structure has been altered slightly at the molecular level in order to change its absorption dynamics.

Autoimmunity A defect in which the body's internal defense system attacks a part of the body itself.

Basal Insulin The continuous flow of insulin designed to offset the liver's gradual secretion of glucose.

Bolus Insulin A burst of insulin designed to act over a short period of time, usually to offset the blood glucose rise that occurs after consuming carbohydrates.

Canula A small, flexible piece of tubing left under the skin once the introducer needle has been removed from an insulin pump's infusion set.

Carbohydrates One of the primary sources of energy found in food; includes sugar, starch, and fiber. Most carbohydrates induce a rapid rise in blood sugar levels.

Complications Harmful long-term effects of diabetes, including eye disease, kidney disease, nerve disease, heart disease, stroke, peripheral vascular problems, gum disease, and joint immobility.

Correction Insulin A quantity of insulin given to bring an elevated blood sugar level down toward normal.

Counter-regulation Bodily secretion of hormones whose effects include the elevation of blood sugar levels and opposition to insulin action.

C-Peptide A portion of the insulin molecule that is broken away soon after insulin is secreted by the pancreas. The level of C-peptide in the blood indicates the amount of insulin being secreted by the pancreas.

Dawn Phenomenon Experienced by most people with and without diabetes, an early-morning increase in blood sugar–raising hormones. In those with diabetes, it can cause an increase in blood sugar levels just before waking.

DCCT Diabetes Control and Complications Trial: A 10-year research study that proved that tight blood sugar control reduces the risk of developing long-term diabetic complications.

Delayed-Onset Hypoglycemia A drop in blood sugar levels that commonly occurs several hours after intense exercise.

Diabetic Ketoacidosis A life-threatening condition in which the body is deprived of insulin, resulting in dehydration and the buildup of acids in the bloodstream.

DKA (see *diabetic ketoacidosis*)

Endocrinologist A physician (MD or DO) who specializes in the treatment of diseases related to glandular problems, such as diabetes.

Fiber A form of carbohydrate that passes through the digestive system intact, without raising blood sugar levels.

Gastroparesis A form of diabetic neuropathy in which food passes through the digestive system at a slower rate than usual.

Glucagon A hormone normally secreted by the pancreas; its primary action is to stimulate the liver to secrete glucose into the bloodstream.

Glucose The form of sugar that circulates in the bloodstream and nourishes most cells of the body.

Glycemic Index A measure of the speed with which food digests and raises the blood sugar level.

Glycogen The compact form in which the liver and muscles store sugar. Counter-regulatory hormones trigger the breakdown of glycogen in order to raise blood sugar levels.

Glycosylated Hemoglobin A measure of the percentage of red blood cells that have glucose stuck to them. This indicates the overall average blood sugar level for the previous 2 to 3 months.

HbA1c (see *glycosylated hemoglobin*)

Honeymoon Phase A period of time, ranging from days to years, after which a person begins taking insulin and still has endogenous (pancreatic) secretion of insulin. Blood sugar levels are generally very stable during the honeymoon phase, and insulin requirements are at relatively low levels.

Hypoglycemia A lower-than-normal level of sugar in the bloodstream.

Hypoglycemia Unawareness A condition in which the body's normal counter-regulatory response to hypoglycemia is blunted; symptoms of hypoglycemia may not appear until the blood sugar level is dangerously low.

Infusion Set The small apparatus used to deliver insulin below the skin by those wearing insulin pumps.

Insulin Analog (see *analog insulin*)

Insulin Resistance A state in which insulin becomes less effective at transporting sugar out of the bloodstream and into the body's cells.

Insulin Sensitivity A state in which insulin's effectiveness at transporting sugar out of the bloodstream and into the body's cells is heightened.

Insulin-to-Carb Ratio A formula used to match the dose of insulin to the amount of carbohydrate being eaten.

Islets of Langerhans Clusters of pancreatic cells which include alpha cells (which secrete glucagon) and beta cells (which secrete insulin).

Ketoacidosis (see *diabetic ketoacidosis*)

Ketones Acid molecules produced during the breakdown of fat. Ketones can accumulate to dangerous levels in the absence of insulin, as the body is unable to break down sugar for fuel.

Lipodystrophy A breakdown of the fat tissue below the skin, resulting in swelling, hardening, or dimpling of the skin and impaired insulin absorption; it is often caused by repeated injections into the same local area of skin.

MDI A program involving multiple daily injections of insulin—typically featuring a basal insulin along with injections of rapid-acting insulin at each meal and snack.

Premixed Insulin A formulation that includes both an intermediate-acting (basal) insulin and a rapid-acting (bolus) insulin in a preset proportion. For example, 75/25 insulin usually consists of 75% intermediate insulin and 25% rapid insulin.

Rebound A counter-regulatory response to hypoglycemia which often results in an unusually high blood sugar level several hours after a low.

Seizure A widespread burst of nervous system activity, usually producing severe, uncontrolled muscle contractions.

Sensitivity Factor The amount that a single unit of insulin lowers the blood sugar level.

Somogyi Phenomenon A rebound (see *rebound,* above) that takes place during sleep.

Sugar Alcohol A "sugar substitute" featuring simple sugars with an alcohol molecule attached to them; this reduces their calorie content and delays their effect on blood sugar levels.

Appendix A

Carbohydrate Factors

MULTIPLY A FOOD'S WEIGHT (in grams) by its factor to determine its carbohydrate content.

Bread & Breakfast

Bagels	0.56
Biscuits	0.47
Bread crumbs, plain	0.70
Bread stuffing	0.18
Corn bread	0.45
Bread, French	0.48
Bread, Italian	0.47
Bread, raisin	0.48
Bread, white	0.47
Bread, whole-wheat	0.39
Croissant, butter	0.43
Croutons	0.68
English muffins	0.33
Pancakes, plain	0.28
Rolls, dinner	0.47
Taco shells	0.54
Waffles	0.36

Candy

Butterscotch	0.95
Caramel	0.75
Fudge	0.78
Hard candies	0.98
Jelly beans	0.93
M&Ms	0.68
Choc. coated nuts	0.44
Choc. coated raisins	0.64
Milk chocolate	0.55
Semisweet chocolate	0.57

Cereal

Crispy Rice	0.87
Cheerios	0.67
Lucky Charms	0.79
Wheaties	0.72
Frosted Mini-Wheats	0.71

All-Bran	0.43
Apple Jacks	0.87
Corn Flakes	0.83
Froot Loops	0.86
Frosted Flakes	0.89
Raisin Bran	0.63
Rice Krispies	0.85
Grape-Nuts	0.72
Shredded Wheat	0.71
Cap'n Crunch	0.82
Quaker Oats & Honey	0.61
Corn Grits	0.12
Cream of Wheat, inst.	0.11
Oats, regular, inst.	0.09
Quaker Oatmeal, inst.	0.14

Combination Foods

Beef Stew	0.14
Chicken pot pie	0.18
Chili with beans	0.07
Coleslaw	0.10
Macaroni & Cheese	0.10
Onion Rings	0.36
Pizza, pepperoni	0.27
Pizza, plain	0.32
Potato Salad	0.09
Shrimp, breaded/fried	0.11
Tuna Salad	0.09
Lasagna	0.16

Condiments/Sauces

Catsup	0.16
Gravy, beef from can	0.04
Hummus	0.08
Salad dressing, Italian	0.10
Syrup, maple	0.67

Tomato paste	0.15
Tomato sauce	0.07

Dairy

Cheddar Cheese	0.01
Cream Cheese	0.02
Mozzarella	0.02
Parmesan, grated	0.03
Ricotta	0.05
Swiss	0.03
Eggs	0.01
Frozen yogurt	0.22
Ice cream, chocolate	0.27
Ice cream, vanilla	0.22
Milk, low fat	0.05
Pudding, chocolate	0.21
Sour cream	0.04

Desserts

Angel food	0.56
Apple pie	0.32
Blueberry pie	0.33
Boston cream pie	0.41
Chocolate cake	0.51
Coffecake	0.44
Cream puffs	0.22
Cupcakes w/ frosting	0.62
Danish, cinnamon	0.43
Doughnut, glazed	0.55
Doughnut, plain	0.48
Eclairs, glazed	0.23
Fruitcake	0.57
Muffin, blueberry	0.45
Pie crust	0.62
Pound cake	0.48
Pumpkin pie	0.24

Sherbet, orange	0.30
Sponge cake	0.60

Drinks

Apple Juice	0.11
Beer, regular	0.03
Beer, light	0.01
Cola	0.10
Cranberry juice	0.14
Daiquiri	0.06
Ginger ale	0.08
Piña Colada	0.22
Wine, sweet	0.11
Wine, dry table	0.01

Fruit and Juices

Apples, raw	0.12
Applesauce, swtnd.	0.18
Applesauce, unswtnd.	0.10
Apricots	0.08
Avocado	0.02
Bananas	0.21
Blackberries	0.07
Blueberries	0.11
Cantaloupe	0.07
Cherries	0.14
Cranberries	0.08
Grapefruit	0.06
Grapes	0.16
Honeydew	0.08
Kiwi	0.11
Mango	0.15
Orange	0.09
Orange w/ peel	0.11
Peaches	0.09
Pears	0.12

Pineapple	0.11
Plums	0.11
Raisins	0.75
Raspberries	0.04
Strawberries	0.04
Tangerines	0.08
Watermelon	0.06

Pasta and Rice

Couscous, cooked	0.21
Egg noodles	0.23
Macaroni	0.27
Spaghetti,	0.26
Rice, brown	0.21
Rice, noodles	0.23
Rice, white	0.27

Snack Food

Almonds	0.14
Almonds, honey rstd.	0.29
Animal crackers	0.73
Beef jerky	0.60
Cashews, dry roasted	0.09
Choc. chip cookies	0.64
Crackers, cheese	0.55
Crackers, matzo	0.80
Crackers, saltines,	0.68
Doritos	0.57
Graham crackers	0.74
Oatmeal cookies	0.65
Peanut butter, smooth	0.13
Peanuts, dry roasted	0.13
Peanuts, Spanish	0.08
Pecans	0.04
Pistachio	0.17
Walnuts	0.07

Oatmeal raisin cookie	0.47	Carrots, raw	0.06
Oreo cookies	0.67	Cauliflower	0.02
Potato chips	0.48	Celery	0.01
Popcorn, air popped	0.62	Corn, sweet	0.16
Popcorn, caramel	0.73	Cucumber	0.01
Popcorn, cheese	0.41	Lettuce	0.01
Popcorn, oil popped	0.47	Mushrooms	0.02
Pretzels	0.76	Onions	0.06
Rice Krispies Treats	0.79	Peas	0.09
Sugar-free cookies	0.57	Peppers	0.04
Tortilla chips	0.57	Pickles, dill	0.02
		Potato, baked	0.22
Vegetables		Potato, French fries	0.27
Artichokes	0.05	Potato, hash brown	0.26
Asparagus, raw	0.02	Potato, mashed	0.15
Beans, baked	0.15	Potato, scalloped	0.08
Beans, kidney	0.16	Spinach	0.01
Beans, lima	0.09	Squash, summer	0.02
Beans, green	0.02	Squash, winter	0.10
Beans, green, soy	0.06	Sweet potato	0.21
Broccoli, raw	0.02	Tomato	0.03
Cabbage	0.03	Yam	0.23

Appendix B

Glycemic Index of Common Foods

A FOOD'S GLYCEMIC INDEX VALUE indicates the speed and ease with which it raises blood glucose levels. Higher numbers indicate a fast, sharp rise in blood sugar. Lower numbers indicate a prolonged, gradual rise in blood sugar.

Bread/Crackers

Bagel	72
Crispbread	81
Croissant	67
French baguette	95
Graham crackers	74
Hamburger bun	61
Kaiser roll	73
Melba toast	70
Pita bread	57
Pumpernickle	51
Rye, dark	76
Rye, light	55
Saltines	74
Sourdough	52
Stoned wheat thins	67
Wheat bread, high fiber	68
White Bread	71

Cakes/Cookies/Muffins

Angel food cake	67
Apple cinnamon muffin	44
Banana bread	47
Banana muffin	65
Blueberry muffin	59
Carrot muffin	62
Chocolate cake	38
Corn muffin	102
Crumpet	69
Cupcake with icing	73

Doughnut	76	Golden Grahams	71
Flan	65	Grape-Nuts	67
Oat-bran muffin	60	Kellogg's	
Oatmeal cookies	55	Mini-Wheats	69
Pound cake	54	Life	66
Scones	92	Oatmeal	49
Shortbread cookies	64	Pancakes	67
Vanilla cake	42	Pop-Tarts	
Vanilla wafers	77	double chocolate	70
		Puffed Wheat	67

Candy

Raisin Bran 73

Cadbury chocolate	49	Rice Bran	19
Dove bar	45	Rice Chex	89
Jelly beans	80	Rice Krispies	82
Lifesavers peppermint	70	Shredded Wheat	69
Lifesavers	70	Special K	66
M&M, peanut	33	Total	76
Mars bar	68	Waffles	76
Milky Way bar	44		
Nestle Crunch	42		

Combination Foods

Skittles	69	Chicken nuggets	46
Snickers bar	40	Fish fingers	38
Twix bar	43	Pizza (cheese)	60
		Sausages	28
		Stuffing	74

Cereals/Breakfast

Taco shells 68

All-Bran	42	
Bran Chex	58	

Dairy

Bran Flakes	74	Chocolate milk	34
Cheerios	74	Custard	43
Cocoa Krispies	77	Ice cream, vanilla	62
Corn Chex	83	Ice cream, chocolate	68
Corn Flakes	83	Milk, skim	32
Cornmeal	68	Milk, whole	27
Cream of Wheat	70	Mousse	31
Crispix cereal	87	Pudding	43
Frosted Flakes	55		

Soy milk	30
Tapioca	81
Yogurt, low fat	33

Fruits & Juices

Apple	38
Apple juice	41
Apricots	57
Banana	55
Cantaloupe	65
Cherries	22
Cranberry juice	68
Dates	103
Fruit cocktail	55
Grapefruit	25
Grapefruit juice	48
Grapes	46
Kiwi	53
Mango	56
Orange	44
Orange juice	52
Papaya	58
Peach	42
Pear	37
Pineapple	66
Pineapple juice	46
Plum	39
Raisins	64
Watermelon	72

Legumes

Baked beans	48
Black beans	30
Blackeyed peas	42
Butter beans	30
Chick peas	33
Fava beans	79
Lentils, red	25
Lima Beans	32
Peas, dried	22
Pinto beans	45
Red kidney beans	19

Pasta

Capellini	45
Fettucini	32
Gnocchi	68
Linguini	55
Macaroni	45
Macaroni & Cheese	64
Noodles, instant	47
Ravioli w/ meat	39
Spaghetti	41
Spaghetti, wheat	37
Spirali	43
Tortellini	50

Powdered Drinks

Nestle hot cocoa	51
Nestle Quik, chocolate	41
Nestle Quik, strawberry	35

Rice/Grain

Brown rice	55
Couscous	65
Instant rice	87
Long grain rice	56
Risotto	69
Vermicelli	58

Snack Foods

Corn Chips	74
Granola bars	61
Kudos bars (choc chip)	61
Nutrigrain bars	66
Peanuts	15
Popcorn	55
Potato chips	54
Pretzels	81
Rice cakes	77
Wheat Thins	67

Soups

Black bean	64
Green pea	66
Lentil	44
Minestrone	39
Split pea	60
Tomato	38

Sports Bars/Drinks

Gatorade	78
Isotar	73
Power Bar, chocolate	58
Sportsplus	74

Sugars & Spreads

Apricot jam	55
Glucose tablets	102
High fructose corn syrup	62
Honey	58
Nutella	33
Strawberry jam	51
Sucrose	64
Syrup, fruit flavored	66

Vegetables

Beets	64
French fries	75
Potato, baked	85
Potato, instant	83
Potato, mashed	91
Potato, boiled	88
Carrots, boiled	49
Carrots, raw	16
Carrot juice	43
Corn	46
Corn, sweet	55
Parsnips	97
Peas	48
Sweet potato	44
Tomato juice	38

Appendix C

Record-Keeping Forms

The record-keeping forms in this section may be downloaded and/or printed from **www.integrateddiabetes.com**

Name:_____

Weekly Diabetes Record

Date:	Breakfast	Snack	Lunch	Snack	Dinner	Snack	Bedtime	Night	Notes
Blood Sugar									
Insulin Dose									
Grams Carb									
Phys. Activity									

Date:	Breakfast	Snack	Lunch	Snack	Dinner	Snack	Bedtime	Night	Notes
Blood Sugar									
Insulin Dose									
Grams Carb									
Phys. Activity									

Date:	Breakfast	Snack	Lunch	Snack	Dinner	Snack	Bedtime	Night	Notes
Blood Sugar									
Insulin Dose									
Grams Carb									
Phys. Activity									

Date:	Breakfast	Snack	Lunch	Snack	Dinner	Snack	Bedtime	Night	Notes
Blood Sugar									
Insulin Dose									
Grams Carb									
Phys. Activity									

Highs:
On-Target:
Lows:

Target Blood Sugar =

+ 1 unit for every _____ points above

− 1 unit for every _____ points below

CARB RATIOS	Breakfast	Lunch	Dinner	Bedtime
Basic Bolus				
w/ Light Exercise				
w/Heavy Exercise				

Date	Time	BS	BS Bolus	Exercise	Carbs	Carb/ExBolus	Total Bolus	Comments

Diabetes Logsheet

Name:_____

Date: _____

	6–7 am	7–8 am	8–9 am	9–10 am	10–11 am	11–12 am	12–1 pm	1–2 pm	2–3 pm	3–4 pm	4–5 pm	5–6 pm	6–7 pm	7–8 pm	8–9 pm	9–10 pm	10–11 pm	11–12 pm	12–1 am	1–2 am	2–3 am	3–4 am	4–5 am	5–6 am
Blood Sugar																								
Grams Carb																								
Insulin																								
Phys. Activity																								
Notes																								

Date: _____

	6–7 am	7–8 am	8–9 am	9–10 am	10–11 am	11–12 am	12–1 pm	1–2 pm	2–3 pm	3–4 pm	4–5 pm	5–6 pm	6–7 pm	7–8 pm	8–9 pm	9–10 pm	10–11 pm	11–12 pm	12–1 am	1–2 am	2–3 am	3–4 am	4–5 am	5–6 am
Blood Sugar																								
Grams Carb																								
Insulin																								
Phys. Activity																								
Notes																								

Date: _____

	6–7 am	7–8 am	8–9 am	9–10 am	10–11 am	11–12 am	12–1 pm	1–2 pm	2–3 pm	3–4 pm	4–5 pm	5–6 pm	6–7 pm	7–8 pm	8–9 pm	9–10 pm	10–11 pm	11–12 pm	12–1 am	1–2 am	2–3 am	3–4 am	4–5 am	5–6 am
Blood Sugar																								
Grams Carb																								
Insulin																								
Phys. Activity																								
Notes																								

Insulin Pump User Logsheet   Name:_____

Date:	6–7 am	7–8 am	8–9 am	9–10 am	10–11 am	11–12 am	12–1 pm	1–2 pm	2–3 pm	3–4 pm	4–5 pm	5–6 pm	6–7 pm	7–8 pm	8–9 pm	9–10 pm	10–11 pm	11–12 pm	12–1 am	1–2 am	2–3 am	3–4 am	4–5 am	5–6 am
Blood Sugar																								
Grams Carb																								
Insulin																								
Phys. Activity																								
Notes (set changes, ketone tests, severe lows, etc.)																								

Date:	6–7 am	7–8 am	8–9 am	9–10 am	10–11 am	11–12 am	12–1 pm	1–2 pm	2–3 pm	3–4 pm	4–5 pm	5–6 pm	6–7 pm	7–8 pm	8–9 pm	9–10 pm	10–11 pm	11–12 pm	12–1 am	1–2 am	2–3 am	3–4 am	4–5 am	5–6 am
Blood Sugar																								
Grams Carb																								
Insulin																								
Phys. Activity																								
Notes (set changes, ketone tests, severe lows, etc.)																								

Date:	6–7 am	7–8 am	8–9 am	9–10 am	10–11 am	11–12 am	12–1 pm	1–2 pm	2–3 pm	3–4 pm	4–5 pm	5–6 pm	6–7 pm	7–8 pm	8–9 pm	9–10 pm	10–11 pm	11–12 pm	12–1 am	1–2 am	2–3 am	3–4 am	4–5 am	5–6 am
Blood Sugar																								
Grams Carb																								
Insulin																								
Phys. Activity																								
Notes (set changes, ketone tests, severe lows, etc.)																								

Appendix D

Carbohydrate Replacement per 60 Minutes of Physical Activity

	Carbohydrate replacement per 60 minutes of physical activity				
	50 lbs (23 kg)	100 lbs (45 kg)	150 lbs (68 kg)	200 lbs (91 kg)	250 lbs (114 kg)
Baseball (practice)	7–10g	14–20g	20–30g	28–40g	35–50g
Basketball	12–15g	24–30g	35–45g	48–60g	60–75g
Bowling	7–10g	14–20g	20–30g	28–40g	35–50g
Boxing (training)	18–22g	37–43g	55–65g	74–86g	92–107g
Carpentry	5–8g	10–16g	15–25g	20–32g	25–40g
Cycling (leisurely)	7–10g	14–20g	20–30g	28–40g	35–50g
Cycling (moderate)	12–15g	24–30g	35–45g	48–60g	60–75g
Cycling (racing)	25–28g	50–56g	75–85g	100–112g	125–140g
Dancing (ballroom)	5–8g	10–16g	15–25g	20–32g	25–40g
Dancing (lively)	8–12g	17–23g	25–35g	34–46g	42–57g
Farming (manual labor)	15–18g	30–36g	45–55g	60–72g	75–90g
Farming (w/power eqpt.)	2–5g	4–10g	5–15g	8–20g	10–25g

Field hockey (practice)	17–20g	34–40g	50–60g	68–80g	85–100g
Football (practice)	17–20g	34–40g	50–60g	68–80g	85–100g
Gardening	7–10g	14–20g	20–30g	28–40g	35–50g
Golf (using a cart)	7–10g	14–20g	20–30g	28–40g	35–50g
Grocery shopping	5–8g	10–16g	15–25g	20–32g	25–40g
Gymnastics	8–12g	17–23g	25–35g	34–46g	42–57g
Handball	15–18g	30–36g	45–55g	60–72g	75–90g
Hiking (w/pack)	10–13g	20–26g	30–40g	40–52g	50–65g
Horseback riding (gallop)	13–17g	27–33g	40–50g	54–66g	67–82g
Horseback riding (trot)	10–13g	20–26g	30–40g	40–52g	50–65g
Horseback riding (walk)	2–5g	4–10g	5–15g	8–20g	10–25g
Housework	3–7g	7–13g	10–20g	14–26g	17–32g
Jogging (3–5 mph)	12–15g	24–30g	35–45g	48–60g	60–75g
Judo/karate (skills practice)	23–27g	47–53g	70–80g	94–106g	117–132g
Machine-tooling	5–8g	10–16g	15–25g	20–32g	25–40g
Mowing (push mower)	13–17g	27–33g	40–50g	54–66g	67–82g
Painting (walls)	7–10g	14–20g	20–30g	28–40g	35–50g
Racquetball	15–18g	30–36g	45–55g	60–72g	75–90g
Raking	5–8g	10–16g	15–25g	20–32g	25–40g
Rowing	13–17g	27–33g	40–50g	54–66g	67–82g
Running (12-min. miles)	13–17g	27–33g	40–50g	54–66g	67–82g
Running (10-min. miles)	20–23g	40–46g	60–70g	80–92g	100–115g
Running (8-min. miles)	28–32g	57–63g	85–95g	104–116g	125–140g
Running (6-min. miles)	38–42g	77–83g	115–125g	154–166g	192–207g
Skating (leisurely)	7–10g	14–20g	20–30g	28–40g	35–50g
Skating (intense)	18–22g	37–43g	55–65g	74–86g	92–107g

Skiing (cross–country)	18–22g	37–43g	55–65g	74–86g	92–107g
Skiing (downhill)	8–12g	17–23g	25–35g	34–46g	42–57g
Soccer (practice)	13–17g	27–33g	40–50g	54–66g	67–82g
Squash	18–22g	37–43g	55–65g	74–86g	92–107g
Swimming (slow)	12–15g	24–30g	35–45g	48–60g	60–75g
Swimming (fast)	22–25g	44–50g	65–75g	88–100g	110–125g
Tennis (doubles)	8–12g	17–23g	25–35g	34–46g	42–57g
Tennis (singles)	18–22g	37–43g	55–65g	74–86g	92–107g
Volleyball (practice)	8–12g	17–23g	25–35g	34–46g	42–57g
Walking (3 mph)	3–7g	7–13g	10–20g	14–26g	17–32g
Walking (4.2 mph)	8–12g	17–23g	25–35g	34–46g	42–57g
Weeding	5–8g	10–16g	15–25g	20–32g	25–40g
Weight training (circuit)	10–13g	20–26g	30–40g	40–52g	50–65g

Acknowledgments

RECOGNIZING THAT CREATIVITY IS nothing more than a modification or improvement on that which already exists, I would like to thank the following groups and individuals for helping build the foundation for *Think Like A Pancreas:*

The original Joslin Philadelphia team (Ann Davin, Kathy Jones, Julie Funk, Bill and Judy Fore) for cultivating my diabetes care skills on a multi-disciplinary level.

Matthew Lore of the Avalon Publishing Group for having the insight to meet the needs of a previously overlooked market.

Dr. Abdul Ghani of Zephyrhills, FL for encouraging me to teach others through the written word.

Drs. Grafton Reeves, Steven Dowshen, and Daniel Doyle and the educational team at A.I. DuPont Hospital for Children in Wilmington, DE for allowing me the opportunity to learn from their fine example.

Drs. Anne Bowen, Alexander Brucker, Gary Carpenter, Austin Chikezie, Barry Goldstein, Serge Jabbour, Lisa Johnson, Cheryl Koch, Christopher Martin, Lina Melhem, Jeffrey Miller, Steven Nagelberg, Nancy Roberts, Judith Ross, Marilyn Ryan, Susan Sandler, Bob Selig, Bruce Stark, Neil Streisfeld, Deebeanne Tavani, Madeleine Weiser, Ned Weiss, and all other physicians in the Philadelphia area who continue to serve their patients well by referring them for diabetes self-management training.

All of my patients who have put their faith in my services despite the lack of cooperation from third party payors.

The staff and volunteers at the Juvenile Diabetes Research Foundation, American Diabetes Association, and Diabetes Exercise & Sports Association for being overworked and underpaid for so long, all for the cause of improving the lives of people with diabetes.

Renee Bernett, the mom of a girl with diabetes, for her tireless efforts in the promotion of diabetes awareness and education.

John Walsh, whose work in type 1 diabetes care and education has set a standard for me to follow.

Marc Blatstein, for getting me started on the right career path.

Everyone at my office (Gina Taddeo, Bret Boyer, Christine Shubin, Joanne Mullin) who worked extra hard so I could write this thing.

My wife Debbie who, for reasons unknown, still supports me in all of my harebrained schemes.

My parents, Paul and Sara Scheiner, who sacrificed more than I ever realized to raise me and my sisters the right way (as a father of four, I can finally understand!).

Index

A

A1c. *See* HbA1c
abdominal obesity, 32
acceptance, 79–81
adolescents
    blood sugar levels in, 158–59
    optimal growth levels of, 13
adrenaline, 176, 211
aerobic exercise, 137–41
    See also exercise
after-meal blood glucose control, 26
aging, 166
air injectors, 57–58
alcohol, 169–70, 186
Allen, Frederick, 20
alternate site testing, 25, 59–60
altitude, 168
American Diabetes Association
    (ADA), 61
anaerobic exercise, 141–42
    See also exercise
analog insulins, 9, 36, 38, 55, 88, 211,
    214
anxiety, 153–54
artificial sweeteners, 44
aspartame (NutraSweet), 44
attitude, 76–81
autoimmunity, 24, 211

B

Banting, Frederick, 20
basal insulin
    action of, 38, 85–88
    defined, 58, 211
    dosage adjustment, 103–20
    fine-tuning, 107–8
    initial doses of, 104–7
    insulin pump therapy and, 110–20
    level, 83–84

peakless, 25
potency of, 35
purpose of, 104
requirements, 84–85, 103–4
testing level of, 113–15
types of, 56
Best, Charles, 20
beta cells, 30
blood glucose meters
    about, 59–60
    accuracy of, 48–49
    companies for, 208
    improvements in, 5–6, 24–25
    initial, 23
blood sugar levels
    anxiety/stress and, 153–54
    bolus insulin doses and, 126–35
    caffeine and, 154–55
    damage from elevated, 11–13
    disease progression and, 155
    factors affecting, 34–48
    factors that lower, 166–69
    factors that raise, 153–66
    fatty foods and, 155–58
    growth and, 158–59
    record keeping/analysis of, 73–76
    regulation of, 33–34
    roller-coaster factors affecting,
        169–74
    secondary influences on, 47,
        153–74
    target ranges for, 53, 185
    timing of dosages and, 148
    weight gain and, 158–59
blood sugar, sources of, 33
blood sugar testing
    accuracy of, 48–49
    alternate sites for, 25, 59–60
    frequency of, 65–66

About the Author

GARY SCHEINER, MS, CDE, is a Certified Diabetes Educator, insulin pump trainer, and exercise physiologist who has written dozens of articles on diabetes, fitness, and motivation. He uses his professional skills and personal experience to teach people the art and science of blood glucose balancing and runs Integrated Diabetes Services, a private practice in Wynnewood, Pennsylvania. Gary can be contacted through his Web site, www.integrateddiabetes.com or by calling 877–735–3648.

The Marlowe Diabetes Library
Good control is in your hands.

MARLOWE DIABETES LIBRARY titles are available from on-line and bricks-and-mortar retailers nationally. For more information about the Marlowe Diabetes Library or any of our books or authors, visit www.marlowepub.com/diabeteslibrary or e-mail us at goodcontrol@avalonpub.com

---

THE FIRST YEAR®—TYPE 2 DIABETES
An Essential Guide for the Newly Diagnosed, 2nd edition

Gretchen Becker | Foreword by Allison B. Goldfine, MD ▪ $16.95

PREDIABETES
What You Need to Know to Keep Diabetes Away

Gretchen Becker | Foreword by Allison B. Goldfine, MD ▪ $14.95

THE NEW GLUCOSE DIABETES REVOLUTION
The Definitive Guide to Managing Diabetes and Prediabetes
Using the Glycemic Index

Dr. Jennie Brand-Miller, Kaye Foster-Powell,
Dr. Stephen Colagiuri, Alan Barclay ▪ $16.95
(Coming Spring 2007)

THE NEW GLUCOSE DIABETES REVOLUTION LOW GI GUIDE TO DIABETES
The Quick Reference Guide to Managing Diabetes Using the Glycemic Index

Dr. Jennie Brand-Miller and Kaye Foster-Powell with Johanna Burani ▪ $6.95

THE 7 STEP DIABETES FITNESS PLAN
Living Well and Being Fit with Diabetes, No Matter Your Weight

Sheri R. Colberg, PhD | Foreword by Anne Peters, MD ▪ $15.95

EATING FOR DIABETES
A Handbook and Cookbook—with More than 125 Delicious, Nutritious Recipes to Keep
You Feeling Great and Your Blood Glucose in Check

Jane Frank ▪ $15.95

TYPE 1 DIABETES
A Guide for Children, Adolescents, Young Adults—and Their Caregivers

Ragnar Hanas, MD, PhD | Forewords by Stuart Brink, MD,
and Jeff Hitchcock ▪ $24.95

KNOW YOUR NUMBERS, OUTLIVE YOUR DIABETES
Five Essential Health Factors You Can Master to Enjoy a Long and Healthy Life
Richard A. Jackson, MD, and Amy Tenderich ■ $14.95

INSULIN PUMP THERAPY DEMYSTIFIED
An Essential Guide for Everyone Pumping Insulin
Gabrielle Kaplan-Mayer | Foreword by Gary Scheiner, MS, CDE ■ $15.95

1,001 TIPS FOR LIVING WELL WITH DIABETES
Firsthand Advice that Really Works
Judith H. McQuown | Foreword by Harry Gruenspan, MD, PhD $16.95

DIABETES ON YOUR OWN TERMS
Janis Roszler, RD, CDE, LD/N ■ $14.95

THINK LIKE A PANCREAS
A Practical Guide to Managing Diabetes with Insulin
Gary Scheiner, MS, CDE | Foreword by Barry Goldstein, MD ■ $15.95

THE ULTIMATE GUIDE TO ACCURATE CARB COUNTING
Gary Scheiner, MS, CDE ■ $9.95

THE MIND-BODY DIABETES REVOLUTION
A Proven New Program for Better Blood Sugar Control
Richard S. Surwit, PhD, with Alisa Bauman ■ $14.95
